The Bliss of Cancer

How I Cured Cancer Naturally,
Lost Weight, And Turned My Life Around.

Evita Ramparte

Edited by Richard S. Gribbin

Cover design and interior design by Natasa Ivancevic and
Shariar Ahmed

LEGAL DISCLAIMER

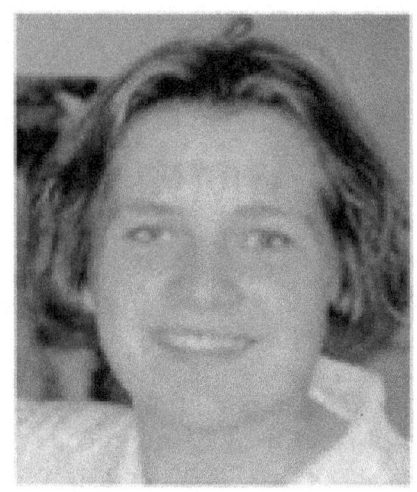 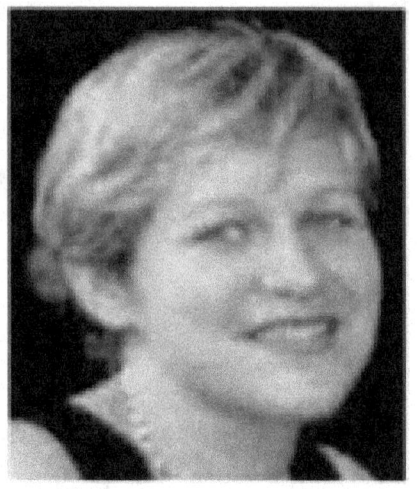

My Transformational Journey

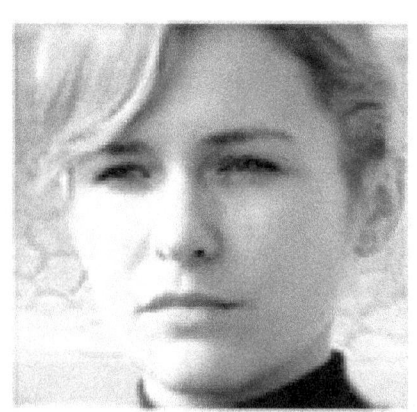 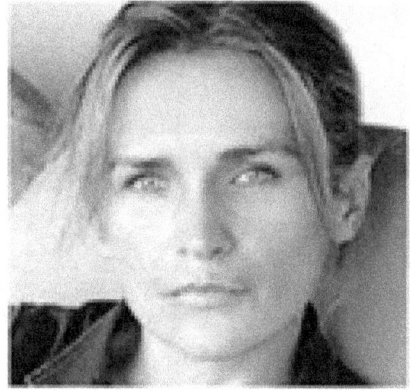

TABLE OF CONTENTS

PREFACE

A lot is done to the female body these days. Her sacred temple is tempered with. Her womb – the holy of holies – is being mutilated, her ovaries and breasts surgically removed. She is discouraged from nursing her babies and forgetting to birth naturally. Ever since Eden, she has been discouraged from eating fruit and cursed to birth in pain...

My story is one of self-awareness and awakening.

A psychic told me something seriously wrong was going on inside my body. Her message saved my life. I have often wondered how my life would have turned out if the doctors had been the first to discover I had cancer. I probably would have bought into the fear they were selling and would have never started fasting and cleansing. I would have just accepted the idea that I was going to die unless I obeyed like a sheep and took all of the medical advice. Well, I was lucky. I didn't give a damn. I could not care less. The message of the psychic healer and her cleansing protocol gave me faith. I just jumped into healing and cleansing, and revamping everything in my life from the inside out. It worked. I wasn't looking back. There was nothing in there for me, and I had nothing to lose. I reclaimed my body and my life.

What I am sharing in this book is purely subjective. It is a reflection of my own experience. I share my story with you the reader because I hope it will spur you to radiant health. Feel free to draw from my experience! But believe nothing; the ultimate test is whether it is working for you. Check with your body, and if it's not working for you, do something else. I invite you to challenge your assumptions, and to test whether you find the ideas contained within helpful for you.

I am thrilled to know that my story is inspiring people all over the world to reclaim their health, their natural beauty, and their inner wisdom. I hear it is awakening them from inside out and empowering to raise like a phoenix from the ashes. I hope to touch as many lives as possible, uplift and raise new leaders on the Earth.

ACKNOWLEDGMENT

My deep thanks go to Nadia for bringing the message of healing into my life, and to my beautiful Mom who never had a chance how to read and write.

How Marriage Nearly Killed Me

It was a cold, muddy winter in Poland. I was opening my eyes with a strong cup of coffee and asking God: "Another day to live? Please stop the train. I am getting off!"

I was married to Brian. It was a hopeless relationship that led to nowhere. I was more of a mother than a wife, in fact, a perfect replica of his mother. Like clockwork, she would call us every Sunday afternoon to run her routine set of questions: "Is Brian eating well? Does he dress nicely? Does he shave?"

Brian was 28 years old, an actor, and a model. Girls would smile at him when we traveled by train. They would say: "I think I know you from somewhere. Haven't I met you before?"

Hearing that, instead of feeling jealous, I would say inside my mind: "Take him. He is yours! I'll pay you!"

Today, I would never date a guy like that, but back than my confidence, self-worth and choice was non-existent. I weighed 183 pounds, and felt as if I was wrapped in a blanket in which someone had made three holes: two to watch television, and one to eat. I was asking, begging, praying, and desperately wanting my life to change. I bought three hair conditioners back then. One coconut, another vanilla, and another I don't remember, maybe it was chocolate. I put the conditioners by the shower curtain, and said to myself, "By the time these conditioners run out, my life will change." I forgot about my secret wish though, and continued to wash my hair each day, as my life silently took on a new course...

I was the breadwinner of our family. I worked as an EnglishPolish interpreter, spending hours, days, and months translating boring legal documents. Brian spent hours, days and months in acting rehearsals, watching movies of James Dean and Marlon Brando, and in the evening we would reunite to watch Star Wars.

During our married life, we had watched Star Wars 66 times. Brian was a fan of Star Wars, ever since the age of five, when he first saw it in a movie theatre and became hypnotized by it. He would buy toys, t-shirts, and anything and everything that had a trace of the unquestioned genius of George Lucas.

Every morning, we would wake up to the Star Wars theme song. Our alarm clock sounded literally like that: *Tam dam dam dam daaaaaaaam... Tam dam dam daaaaaaaaaaam dam... Tam dam dam daaaaaaaaaam.* It was the symphony of John Williams, the soundtrack to warp speed and all things Jedi.

Besides Star Wars toys, Brian also had a large comic book collection. Twenty thousand comic books were stored at his parents' New York home: the first Spiderman, the first Batman, the first Mickey Mouse, and Donald Duck. His comic book collection was estimated to be worth at least two hundred thousand dollars. Despite this wealth of collectibles, we lived in a little studio, on the top floor of an old post-communist apartment block. Without insulation, the winters were freezing cold and the summer heat was unbearable. Everything I was earning paid for rent, food, and his toys. At home, we had the figures of Master Yoda, Han Solo, Princess Leia, Luke Skywalker, Darth Vader, the Imperial Guards, and star-ships. We were only missing Jabba the Hutt.

Meanwhile, I prayed. I prayed that something would change in my life. It didn't feel right to leave. It didn't feel right to stay.

Poor Brian, I was thinking. How would he manage without me?

I was stuck. They say: 'Marriage is a wonderful institution.' But, who wants to live in an institution. Mine certainly was.

Every single day I was called "stupid" by my husband, and there was not a "stupid-free" day in the three years of my married life. I was cooking, cleaning, making money, pumping up his confidence, and working as his acting manager. I was booking his auditions, and providing sex. One by one he would flunk every audition. And sex? He would flunk that, too.

Divorce was on my mind, since the very day I married, or more precisely, since the wedding night. Our sex was painful, obligatory, awful, boring, purely physical, abusive, and humiliating. I simply felt used. He would just climb on me, do his thing and turn around and go to sleep. My girlfriends would talk about sex with so much laughter, and I kept wondering, what's so fun about sex? It hurts! Or at best, I feel nothing. My mother raised me as a good Catholic girl. I was told my husband would respect me if I were a virgin. Poor thing. I saved myself to get this. Sex had no flavor to me. It felt as if I was drinking wine, but all I tasted was water.

I had no boyfriend when I was a teenager. I wasn't someone's high-school sweetheart. I was a chubby girl, with pimples on my face, and pimples on my back that no one knew about. Ever since I entered grade school, I had kept gaining weight that I couldn't seem to lose. School felt a bit like pushing a circle into a square, so I guess I gained weight because of stress. Kids laughed at me when I was doing sports. Mom bribed our family doctor to write me a permanent excuse from swimming lessons, because she saw someone drown when she was young. So I didn't learn to swim as a child and I wasn't moving much during my school years. When they were picking teams for basketball or volleyball, they would always pick me last. I remember I was standing there alone and I could see them roll their eyes when they had to choose me. Running was the worst. For some reason, my entire school found it entertaining when I was running. Maybe because my score was the worst in history.

In high school, every guy I liked was snatched up by one of my girlfriends before he ever noticed me. How could he? I was fat. I was wrapped in a thick, man-repelling blanket of bloat. Today, I know my body was actually swollen and inflamed. Back then, I called it fat. Nothing much happened between me and the boys in high school. A kiss maybe. I was a 23-year-old virgin when I married Brian.

And sex with Brian was so painful—both physically and emotionally—that I did everything I could to avoid it. My best tactic was to have guests all the time! Lots of dinners, and movie nights with friends. I loved it when they would stay and sleep over. I kept having a headache. Those horrible migraine attacks came in really handy. And I even got us a little kitten, a black and white tiny creature we ironically named Myszka (mouse in Polish). The kitten was a great diversion!

As a last resort, I learned how to give oral sex. At least then, I didn't have to deal with the pain of him entering my body.

At least once a week Brian would tell me that I would be nothing without his family. They were middle class Polish immigrants who suspected I married for money. A bitter accusation. I had no idea where this mysterious money was. Brian obviously had low self-esteem, and seemed to hope that if he put me down enough, somehow his value would rise.

All of this: the guilt, the blame, and the shame—they were the three shades of judgment that blended together to turn my life into one long, gray, shady day. These poisonous emotions kept me stuck like a butterfly in a spider's web. I cried for change. I wanted out. My soul, my body and my spirit wanted out. The only thing that cheered me up was food...

How a Psychic Saved My Life

Everything changed on the eve of the New Millennium. The year 2000! We were celebrating with friends. One of the guests had a message for me that later on would save my life.

She sat straight, spoke softly and carried herself with a lot of dignity. Her name was Nadia. She was from Ukraine. I never met her before and never saw her again.

She must have been observing me during our house party, since she seemed to know a lot about me right when we met.

"You have pain in your lower back. Do you want me to fix it? I am a chiropractor," she offered kindly.

I accepted with enthusiasm and gratitude. I was proud that I knew what a chiropractor was. I had a previous spinal adjustment when I was living in Israel.

We left the party and went up to the attic. She scanned my body with her hands, looked intensely into my eyes and around me, as if looking for something. She adjusted my spine with a sound of cracking, and then said:

"You have sixteen stones in your gallbladder. Your pancreas is weak. You crave sugar during the day, and if you don't eat something sweet, you feel like you're about to faint, right?"

Yes, I admitted. How did she know? I was a sugar junkie, living on Coke and Snicker bars every day.

I always craved sugar around 11 a.m. and again between 3-4

p.m. Otherwise, my legs would become so weak that I felt as if I was about to pass out on the street.

She waved her left hand over my body, up and down, and continued to scan me with her piercing eyes. She wasn't interested in making friends, which disappointed me. Rather, she behaved like a detective investigating a case, searching for the cause of my condition.

"You have something serious going on with your reproductive organs," she finally pronounced.

"You must go to a gynecologist and get tested."

Ok. I will, I promised both to her and to myself. I knew something had been eating me. I had even mentioned it to Brian.

"You have to do a cleanse," she added. "You will need to have an enema morning and evening. You will rise early, and go to sleep before nine. For three days you will go on a juice fast. You will drink apple juice every two hours, and you will drink olive oil and lemon juice twice in the afternoon. You will not eat anything at all in this time."

She was so serious about it that she actually handed me a sheet of paper and made me take notes. I was thinking she was mad. As in crazy. Me? Not eating? I could imagine for an hour or so … but a whole day? Three whole days? What? I would die if I did that!

She gave me lengthy instructions about juicing, detoxifying the body, digestion and nutrition, and she told me to get an enema bag. I took notes out of politeness, but I wasn't thinking I was going to apply this outlandish advice.

I was sincerely thinking she was crazy. The enema idea seemed especially nuts. Putting a tube up my butt? Inserting some coffee? Coffee into the butt? OK. What else? I was getting impatient at this point and was hoping to get this meeting over soon, and go back to my friends to party.

"It's powerful. A way to cure cancer," she added. "Don't stop fasting until you get all sixteen stones out of your gallbladder."

Yeah, right.

We walked down and joined the celebration. The next day, when saying good-bye, Nadia looked at Brian, and said to me:

"Don't worry. Everything will be all right. Do what is necessary."

I knew Nadia saw what was coming. Did she know that if I did the cleanse, nothing would stop me from freedom?

By then, I had threatened Brian with divorce too many times. As a result, the subject matter lost any impact. I was the girl crying wolf (that I was going to leave), but those were only attempts to gain some respect for myself. What did I win by doing that? A deal that he would take the trash out, or vacuum the place once a week?

Once we got the kitten, I actually started to consider moving out and renting my own apartment, but then I didn't know what to do about the pet. Who would take her? Me or him? How to find an apartment with an owner who would tolerate the pet? And, of course, all these questions were nothing but excuses.

But the day I met Nadia, Mouse, our black and white kitten, solved that problem for me by deciding to leave. She jumped out of the balcony at my parents' house, and died tragically on the concrete. Although I was very sad, I was also grateful to her. She freed me. As soon as I returned to Warsaw, I went to the doctor. The gynecologist was accompanied by his assistant. They did an ultrasound and nearly shouted at me:

"Where are your ovaries!?" they asked.

What? I didn't understand. "Where are your ovaries?" They looked at me with scared faces.

"You have such large tumors that we can't see your ovaries any more. How could you walk? Pick up things? Have sex?"

I had been feeling pain in my abdomen, but I had not paid attention to it. My married life was centered on Brian. He was the Star. He was our running horse in the race—our champion. He deserved all the attention.

The doctors told me to come back and get tested. They said I might have cancer. It was obvious, and Nadia was right. Indeed, exactly as she said, I did have "something serious going on with my reproductive system". No wonder intercourse was so painful! And, she saw it without all that expensive equipment doctors have. I wasn't going to wait. On the way home, I went to the farmers' market and got all the stuff I needed for the juicing protocol: beets, apples, lemons. I got the extra virgin olive oil, which nearly broke my budget. I visited at least three different pharmacies to find an enema bag. I hand-carried all the shopping bags home.

"The doctors say I might have cancer. I am going for the test tomorrow," I announced as soon as I got home. I was kind of excited for the sensation this would create. I was hoping finally Brian's world would start spinning around me.

"You will be fine. Don't worry about it!"

He waved his hand, and flipped the channels on the television.

What? Not even a hug? I was shocked. My eyes opened wide and I kept blinking. He paid no attention, and I was attention starved.

I silently cried in the kitchen, overwhelmed by doubts: is this the same guy that I've been taking care of all these years? Cruising back and forth, bedroom-kitchen-bedroom, every time he had a fever? His reaction was like a wake-up call. I dried my tears, took a deep breath, gathered myself, and I decided to live.

I had no idea then that Brian had just given me the best advice in the world, and that he would be my greatest teacher. Paradoxically, he was right. I was going to be fine, and I was not going to worry about it.

Today, I can say with gratitude: he saved my life! If I had received love and attention from him at this critical moment of my life—just because of cancer—I probably would have chosen to stay sick for years, and die slowly in his arms. After all, I was starved for love.

I didn't get the dope, the fix, the drug of his love and attention that I so desperately needed.

Instead, I shook off fear, doubt, guilt, blame, regret, resentment, sorrow, sadness, suffering, shame and every-thing else, and I swore to myself:

All right! From now on, my life is in my own hands. I am responsible for one life. My own!

How Doctors Nearly Killed Me

I returned to my doctors for test results after my three-day cleanse.

I felt so great in my body, and so differently that I knew the tests they did on me last week were completely irrelevant.

I had undergone a profound inner surgery. My body felt so great. I felt slimmer, lighter, younger. My mind was barely catching up with the change. I just knew that if I continued on this path I would become a really healthy beauty.

I entered the office radiant, joyful and optimistic. I brought the notes I took with Nadia and I was going to share with them all my newly discovered cleansing secrets. I was bubbling over with excitement, and eager to tell them that I felt great. That I had just passed sixteen gallbladder stones, or maybe even twenty. I wanted to share that the gallstones were like lentils, but softer because I drank apple juice and olive oil. And that I passed colon stones, too. They were like walnuts. It was gross. It smelled like sewage, but I felt great.

I smiled a hello, and showed them my loose pants around my waist.

"We are very sorry," they announced with long faces. "The results are positive. You have cancer."

I kept smiling, and kept to my own agenda. I needed to tell them what I did so they would tell their patients. I was naive. The conversation went more like I was a Jehovah's Witness trying to convert some Hari Krishnas.

The doctors expected me to follow a standard protocol that they hand out to cancer patients. I was to show up next day at the hospital, with my pajamas and a tooth-brush. They had everything ready for me. Outlined. Except... I was no sheep. I asked too many questions. Eventually, they got upset with me for not being a good girl. They said they wouldn't treat me in the future, unless I would obey them now. I asked:

"Excuse me, Gentlemen. Do you know the cause of my disease?"

They laughed at me:

"We'd get a Nobel Prize if we knew the cause of cancer." "Really?" I paused for a moment. "So why would I listen to you about the solution?"

I didn't get a Nobel for my "Privately Sponsored Cancer Research", but I already knew what two things caused it for me: toxic food and toxic thinking. I decided to give myself some time and continued to cleanse, eat healthily and clarify my relationships so that I would be happy. I told them I would come back healthy in a few months, and if not, I could always go for the surgery or chemotherapy.

One thing helped. I remembered a really great biology teacher in grade school. She had told us that if a lake has been poisoned by a factory nearby, it is enough for the factory to be shut down and the lake will purify itself over a period of time. That gave me faith that my body would do exactly the same. I decided to continue to cleanse, and see what would happen.

I monitored my tumors on ultrasound every two to three weeks. I went to a different clinic for that, since I didn't want to make the gynecologists who had diagnosed me with ovarian cancer even angrier. I just needed a regular checkup. I continued eating healthily: no dairy, no sugar, no meat, no bread, no white rice, no refined wheat. No. No. No. I went through my kitchen cupboard and cleared out everything that had a trace of white sugar (didn't know ketchup had a ton!) or dairy, and eggs (mayonnaise!).

My taste buds changed during the cleanse, so I craved fruit, fruit, and fruit, as well gentle leafy greens with tomatoes and cucumbers, vegetable soups, steamed veggies, and I stayed away from meat. In fact, meat seemed dead when I tasted it.

I made a big basket of "toxic goodies" and gave it to the homeless. I continued juicing and eating everything that was alive. I ate no fat – zero. No animal fat or plant based fat – no seeds, nuts, avocados or oils. I overate on fruit. I never starved myself. It was my cravings that changed, healed and discovered a pleasure of fruit which felt like returning back to Eden.

Four months later, I was 83 pounds lighter, and cancer-free. My friends didn't recognize me. I had to stop people on the street. They would look into my eyes and shout with amazement: "It's you!?"

My doctors weren't happy at all. My victory somehow meant to them that they lost on the playing field. So sad. They were not invested in my healing! It seemed as if they had spent years and money for an expensive medical school education and now stood stubbornly defending its philosophies at all costs, even if it made no sense.

I told them I quit two things: toxic food and toxic thinking. To my disappointment, they weren't interested in learning how I had gotten well. They belittled my success. They said that I must have taken steroids.

Today, I wonder what would have happened to me, how my life would have turned out if I had actually listened to the doctors and gone for the surgery. If I had survived the illness and the treatment, I would probably have been an obese, depressed woman; quite possibly infertile and, most certainly, dumb.

Today, when I talk with doctors about how my cancer disappeared naturally, they almost always say that I must have been misdiagnosed. Interesting. So, if I had been misdiagnosed and operated on and chemo/radiated for no reason, then that would somehow be okay? I wonder how many women have that happen to them? Is that the norm? And, what happens to them next? How many women with endometriosis are send for chemo today? Is the system outperforming? Is it on set on overkill?

Somehow, in our culture it is possible for the medical professionals to make a mistake (and oops, by the way, then you are really screwed), but there is no space for the patient to have a healing victory.

How about this idea: a victory party of no more cancer that would be celebrated together with his or her doctor? How cool would that be?!

Over and over I meet people who have been treated with surgery, chemotherapy, and/or radiation. They lost their hair, their teeth, their strength and their beauty. Their immune system is shattered.

Some financial analysts say: "The pharmaceutical industry is making more money on drugs that remove the side effects of chemotherapy than from chemotherapy itself."

Whenever oncologists gather, the word cure rarely crosses the lips. The dialogue, as we can read in the Journal of American Medical Association, centers on prolonging the patient's life for at least five years from the diagnosis. Some of the cancer patients survive beyond five years after chemo treatments. If they do— Wow!—they are considered absolute cancer survivors, and— Wow! Bravo!—the medical community is proud to announce we beat cancer. And yet the bulk of them die like flies soon after the fifth year.

Not surprisingly. Only thirty minutes of class time is given to the study of nutrition at medical colleges across America. And this treatment of nutrition as a non-issue is the exact point where doctors sever themselves from the teachings of Hippocrates— widely held to be the Father of Western Medicine—who stated, "Let food be thy medicine, and medicine be thy food".

Indeed, although nearly 98% of modern doctors take some watered-down version of a Hippocratic Oath, its main premise, as stated in the original version: "First, do no harm", has been long removed from the oaths of today, and that idea itself apparently abandoned.

Instead of following in Hippocrates' ancient footsteps, medical students spend their youth studying pathology—which literally means "the study of suffering"—learning to recognize thousands of symptoms, and then learning about the thousands of drugs that suppress the symptoms deeper into the body. The practice seems as insane as memorizing a telephone directory.

And leads right to the news now going mainstream, as reported in the May 2014 issue of the highly respected Consumer Reports magazine, which takes no advertising and therefore maintains a non-biased stance of independent research. The article, entitled Survive Your Stay at the Hospital reports that 440,000 deaths each year are due to medical errors. That's more than 1,000 per day, and more than half the deaths that occur in U.S. hospitals each year. From errors. And food at the hospital is so bad that it has earned a joke: "If you want to get sick, go eat at the hospital."

Given that fact, my cancer healing story borders on resurrection. Whenever I share this chapter of my life with Western audience, people look at me as if I have risen from the grave. Cleaned up pretty well, I would say. Two months after I completely healed I was first time ever photographed in a modeling shoot. That was a big change – from an ugly duckling into a swan!

How I Reclaimed My Life

So what did I do that caused my cancer to disappear and my knee to heal? What was the cleanse that saved my life?

Day One. Enema, right in my butt. *You've got to be kidding me!* I thought to myself, while inserting the tube.

It was Friday morning, 6 a.m. I began my cleanse.

My husband was sleeping, unaware of my conspiracy in the bathroom. God forbid he would enter and see me with a hose of coffee water dripping into my butt! I told myself: *Why not? What have I got to lose?* I didn't need to calculate. This was not about trying. I was doing it. I was moving forward like the Mongolian army. No option of going back and hesitating. I was going to WIN this battle or die.

Going to a filthy Polish hospital would have meant a risk of getting even sicker. News stories about people catching staph infections were abundant on TV. Visiting a private clinic was too much of a luxury. Only former communist politicians could afford it.

Looking back, I think I was protected by some unseen force.

I had no choice but to heal myself by relying on nature. I followed Nadia's instructions precisely. After all, she was correct in her diagnosis. With her sonar vision, she saw something that doctors had detected only by using highly sophisticated equipment. And, she had no vested interest in doing so!

How could I not trust her? What option did I have? So there I was, in my bathroom, before the dawn of a new day; with a mysterious enema bag hanging from the shower door; resting my knees on an old beach towel and breathing in deeply while a lukewarm liquid of filtered water with coffee in it was dripping into my gut with a hope of producing some kind of miracle.

Strange. No one I knew would ever do that kind of stuff. Not even my mom, my grandma; no one in my family. I called my girlfriends, and found that many of them had ovarian cysts, tumors, fibroids, etc. They all considered it normal, and they were not alarmed by it at all. They just had a surgery and it was gone. One of my friends lost an ovary when the scalpel slipped. That is a 50% less chance of having a baby, I thought to myself. But, maybe she didn't want to have children. I did. I knew that one day I would give birth to a child.

Niagara Falls. That is what it felt like, when I first released the liquid out of my bowels. I nearly puked. My belly became full and for a split second all I could see was black in my head. I had to stop, sit on the toilet and release. Lucky I didn't spill it on the floor. Shit! I cursed silently, from the gut of my mind.

I recalled the Ukrainian lady preparing me for that. Be calm.

It's OK. Refill the bag, kneel down and flush in and flush it out! Use the entire solution, until the pot is empty.

I prayed not to wake up Brian. He had no idea what I was doing. Well, neither did I! I could just imagine the look on his face if all of a sudden he opened the door and saw me kneeling on the floor with a long tube in my butt. That made me smile.

I used up about two gallons of coffee liquid, and when the pot was empty I showered, and was actually surprised with the rush of new energy in my body. The enema made me feel light and awake. It made me feel so good!

Although when I entered the kitchen, I wondered: three days without food!? How am I going to make it? That sounds Crazy! A day without coffee, without Snicker bars, or Coke? It was hard to imagine. Without a cream-cheese sandwich with ham, without the yogurt, cereal, pasta or rice? What's wrong with that? Why not?

I had doubts. But strangely, I was not hungry.

I threw fresh apples into the juicer, and drank two glasses, gulping it down. I felt it streaming down my throat and into my digestive tract, which had just been somewhat emptied. Chills went down my body. It made me cold. Two hours later, I juiced again. Nadia had told me to stay home, and rightly so. I was on the toilet with diarrhea, just when my husband woke up. It was 9 a.m. and seemed like the middle of the day for me. I was bright awake. Just shaking with shivers. I cleaned the bathroom and let him in.

The more juice I drank, the dizzier I felt. Drinking the juice loosened something inside me. At noon, I prepared a mixture of olive oil and lemon juice. A horrible fifty-fifty solution. It tasted like salad dressing, but where was the salad? I shook it up in the jar, and kept staring at the mixture with bubbly oil dancing behind the glass. I cannot possibly drink that! I swallowed a bit, and spit it out into the sink. What the hell am I doing?!

I got angry. I was angry with that woman from Ukraine, Nadia. I asked Brian to turn on Star Wars music and crank it up really loud, so that I would not hear my thoughts. Tam dam dam dam dam dam. I needed John Williams' music to inspire my inner Jedi. I drank half! My taste buds indicated their disgust. Tam dam dam dam dam. I swallowed the rest of it. My head turned circles, I felt dizzy. I leaned against the counter and waited for it to go down. It did, and I suddenly felt very sleepy.

Nadia was right to prepare me for all the chills, the ups and downs, the shivers and hot flashes. She said: it is like an internal surgery on your body. At least I knew that what was happening was normal, and that I had to allow it. I took a nap, and woke up for another shot of salad dressing without a salad, just to find out that the toilet cannot be occupied while I am doing this. I knocked on the door desperately. My head felt dizzy. This time, I had both diarrhea and vomiting. I remembered my mother, how she used to hold my head when I would throw up as a child. There was no one to hold my head this time. Vomiting and convulsions were shaking my body.

4 p.m. and 6 p.m. I was allowed to have more juice. It just made me go to the bathroom more. I took a book to read in the toilet, as it seemed most of my day would be spent there. Useless though. My eyesight was too blurry for me to be able to read; my head was spinning. At 7 p.m. I had an enema again, and I also had enough. I immersed my body in a salt bath, and nearly fell asleep in the bathtub.

This was the first day of my cleanse. I had no idea what I was doing, and no idea why. It was an experiment. Some-thing I had never done. Something no one I knew ever did. I wondered if it made any sense. The water got cold and I opened my eyes. I put my slippers on, and fell asleep like a baby. It was barely eight o'clock. I forgot to take my robe off.

Day Two. I woke up again at 5 a.m. Going to sleep early and rising early, according to Nadia, was supposed to help my liver to purify my blood.

All right. Here we go, the same routine. I barely opened my eyes. The coffee enema woke me up. Apple juice every two hours, and the disgusting olive oil drink at noon, and then more apple juice. Making me feel dizzier, shittier, and just plain yucky!

I was sick and tired of it. It really felt like an internal surgery, and I was about to give up. The sugar junkie, the coffee addict, the carnivore—all of them at once were refusing to collaborate. I walked around home feeling cold shivers, and feeling angry! I felt deprived of the things I liked, things that were normal to me, my everyday life. Brian was watching his movies, doing his acting rehearsals, and didn't give a damn.

I was furious. Why did he not care? Why did he not feel sorry for me? I was frustrated that I had to do this cleanse. I was impatient. I had to dig the tunnel even though I saw no light.

Nadia had prepared me for these emotions.

She had mentioned something about feeling sad, and afraid, and upset. I had not paid much attention to this. Now, I felt all the anxiety running through me up and down, and I could not pacify it with any food. I just could not sweep it under the rug any more. Fear kept staring at me from every corner of my life!

I had to face it. I didn't like my feelings. I did not like my body. I did not like anything. I was not even hungry at this point.

I had a terrible headache, shivers and I felt deprived. Like a spoiled brat!

It was on the evening of Day Two when I realized why cleansing and fasting made sense.

During my evening enema routine, my stones started to come out! It seemed as if the apple juice loosened my internal tissues enough to open them up. The olive oil lubricated the digestive tract for the gallstones to soften up, slip out and pass through, with no pain. Each time I filled my gut with the coffee liquid, the water was literally picking up the stones and passing them out—into the toilet. Worst of all, Nadia had told me to count them! She instructed me to put a big soft plastic strainer between the toilet seat and my butt, and catch them!

The stench was horrible. It smelled like the city sewage system. Sulfur! I closed my nose and took a closer look. The gallbladder stones looked a bit like lentils. There were also colon stones, which looked like walnuts. I had no idea I carried so much junk inside my gut!!

Nadia said I had to do a spiritual assignment during my cleanse. She told me: make a list of everything you say good-bye to. Cool! I wrapped myself in my warm wool blanket, and poured it all out. Everything. The entire story I had been carrying around. That was an emotional diarrhea. It seemed that my mind was also passing out stones. I felt relieved then, even though I also felt some-what responsible for choosing all that drama.

I didn't realize yet that since I had allowed all that crap, I could just as well have chosen something great. I was afraid to leave Brian. I was afraid I was going to be alone and nobody would want me. I knew this cleanse meant divorce. Nothing less. It meant we would grow apart, and it was just a matter of time before the bubble would come to the surface.

On Day Three, I felt extremely weak. It all made sense though. I was about to become the Enema Queen. I discharged even more stones. One more day on dazzling apple juice and the bittersweet lemon-olive oil concoction.

This time, it went smoothly through me, in and out. I would gulp a glass and humbly make my trip into the bathroom. I would sit on the toilet, and read a book about cleansing and nutrition that Nadia recommended to me. It opened my eyes. All the whys were in there. The cause and effect. (And what those doctors couldn't answer.) What we eat and why we slowly die. This process is caused by stress and the effect is disease. As the author described it, what we eat can result in a slow death instead of giving us life. So true; I hadn't felt like I was really living.

My mind cleared out. Somehow, an inner silence occurred within me. In the evening of Day Three, I was very glad that I had fasted and gone through the cleanse. I said good-bye to all the stones, both the physical and the emotional ones. That night, I knew my life would never be the same again. I still felt too weak to determine the course of it. I just knew I was free to choose a different way.

Later that same night, when I washed my face in the bathroom, it felt as if the tap water slowed down and spoke to me. It whispered to me with sweet voices. I must be insane, I thought. I rinsed my face and looked into the mirror. My skin cleared, and eyes shined brightly. I began to see the real me emerge. I felt light, I felt relieved, and I went to sleep with gratitude. I knew life will never be the same. Only one thought was now on my mind: Thank you! Thank you! Thank you!

How Fasting Can Be Fun

So you are probably asking yourself: How can I undergo this transformation from the inside out? How can I reclaim my life?

Let me guide you. Let me hold your hand.

Ready?

First, let me ask you a brutal question: Have you suffered enough? Or, perhaps you'd like to suffer more? How about another ten or fifteen years? If so, please put this book away, and pick it up in ten or fifteen years, ok? I feel obliged to warn you. If you apply what I am about to share, your life will never be the same. Your body will change, your mind will open up, and your relationships will be effected as you will no longer be willing to hold onto the same crap that everyone else does. You will get out of the limited reality built for you to fit. You will grow bigger, and it will no longer be comfortable.

OK. I have warned you. Now, if you are still holding this book open, let's start!

Fasting is going to be your vehicle for healing, cleansing and ultimately, changing your life. Fasting is purging for your body and it is also a rite of passage for your insane mind to get out of the way, surrender and acknowledge that you are in charge.

Your mind is insane, did you know that? It's absolutely cuckoo!!

It likes to doubt you, criticize you, and sabotage you. If the mind is intelligent, why does it do that? Isn't it here to serve you? If the mind is so smart, why is it not happy, and why does it create disease?

So, let's conquer your insane mind, let's get it out of the way, and make you thrive! You will be surprised to find out the key is fasting!

• How Does Fasting Work?

My friend Len Watson is the Master-Faster of Hawaii. He has 36 years of experience in the raw vegan lifestyle. He eats super healthily, and regularly fasts a couple of times each year. Here's what Len says about fasting:

"Fasting is the oldest, safest, therapeutic method of healing the body, mind and spirit. Fasting can be something that nothing else is. There is no replacement for it. You can take cleansing supplements, cleansing foods, but fasting is non-doing. It is getting out of the way, and letting the body come into homeostasis and balance."

Len continues: "We have about 40-60 trillion cells in our bodies. Out of those, 50% are in peak condition, 25% are new cells, and 25% are old cells. During fasting the body eats up the old cells, recycles the amino acids, and makes protein. This way, it creates more room for new cells, and stimulates their production— especially in the brain. Nothing can regenerate and rejuvenate like fasting. No supplement. No herb."

When you are fasting, your body goes into a state of autolysis (self-digestion). It eats up itself! How cool is that? It releases very strong enzymes that eat up the toxic stuff, everything that's no longer useful; and as a result, you feel lighter, you feel more space and you have more energy.

Really? No Food?

To assist in this process I will not confuse my body by eating. Once the body kicks in the process of autolysis, it doesn't like to be thrown back and forth into consumption and digestion. I may prepare my body by eating vegan meals for at least a week before, and eating smaller portions. I may also do a three-day fast before I choose to fast for seven days or longer.

When I am fasting I make sure no solid food crosses my lips whatsoever. Not even one bite. It's a matter of communication with my body. I know that when I take a bite, soon after I will take another, and another, and before I know I am eating, and the fast is over. Food stimulates digestion. As soon as it enters the mouth, information goes out into the stomach to release the digestive enzymes. That means we are eating!

There is nothing wrong with eating. I love eating. Just not when I am fasting. It's like fire and ice - they don't mix. Either we are cooling, or we are heating.

Cellular Nutrition

When I fast on raw organic juices, or coconut water, I discover that tons of nutrients will feed my body on a cellular level. That means my body will be feasting while I am fasting. I make sure I super-hydrate by drinking a lot of liquid!

I will have cravings for food now and then. Every couple of days I may have a crisis, and may feel like all of a sudden I can't live without grandma's apple pie or that slice of pizza. I ask if it is truly what my body requires at the moment, or is it an emotional craving, a memory of my mind, or maybe... something to forgive?

Although at any time I am free to break the fast and start eating, is it what I really would like to do? What if I open a coconut or drink a glass of freshly pressed juice, and my cravings are gone?

What if I am actually thirsty when I believe I am hungry?

I walk through the supermarket and look at all the crap they sell in flashy packaging, and it doesn't do a thing for me. I can totally live without it. It can cease existing. I can eat it, and I don't have to. I have a choice, and I choose not to.

I have friends and clients who overcame addictions and discovered they can thrive without tobacco, drugs, and alcohol, because they learn about the power of choice by choosing to thrive without food altogether, for a set period of time.

• Vision Quest

Fasting makes my blood alkaline, and as a result my mind is sharp and at my service, my body is more inclined to move and dance, and my whole being is in a natural state of gratitude and joy.

I fast several times a year. Not only because my body likes it. Above all, I fast for the clarity of vision that fasting creates. Fasting naturally releases DMT in the brain (linked to visionary and self-transcendent experiences). It expands my being, and gives me a sense of inner knowing. It is a trans-dimensional experience working on the physical and etheric aspects. No wonder that so many holy people received their key visions during a period of fasting!

If you look into the history of humankind, all the greatest prophets and spiritual leaders fasted. Jesus fasted for 40 days, and even though he was tempted by the Devil, he refused to eat, and said: "It is not only with bread that man finds sustenance, but with every word of God." Saint Peter, Saint Paul, and my favorite heroine, Mary Magdalene, also fasted!

Buddha fasted and meditated by the Bodhi Tree, and he reached Enlightenment. Prophet Muhammad was literally addicted to fasting, praying and bowing down to God. He fasted more than just the month of Ramadan. Saint Francis, one of the greatest heroes of Christianity, always fasted whenever he needed guidance, as well as many other mystics.

Prof. Arnold Ehret, in his book on 'Rational Fasting for Physical, Mental and Spiritual Rejuvenation', published in 1926, states:

"All so-called miracles of the saints have their only origin in ascetics, and are today impossible but for the simple reason that, although much praying is done, no fasting is adhered to. This is the only solution of this quarrel. We have no more miracles because we have no more saints, i.e. sanctified and healed by ascetics and fasting."

Many founding fathers of the American Republic practiced fasting and were vegetarian, such as Benjamin Franklin, who wrote: "The best of all medicines is resting and fasting." Gandhi announced he was beginning a "fast unto death" in protest of caste separation. Hundreds of Tiananmen students fasted in protest against the Chinese government. Lady Diana used to fast, and God knows who else!

Whenever I find myself stuck and overwhelmed by the density of this world, I stop doing whatever I am doing, I turn off all electronics, I retreat, and go fasting for at least three days. It opens me up for receiving solutions that are beyond the radar of my cleverness. The events that are unleashed as a result of this process always turn out to be all about ease, joy and glory, and sometimes even bordering on what people could call a miracle.

A miracle is just a point of view. In America, when I say my cancer disappeared from cleansing and fasting, people look at me as if I just resurrected from the grave. In Poland, most of my friends know that if you are sick, you've got to cleanse, and you will be fine. Nobody considers it a miracle. In the words of Prof. Arnold Ehret: "During the Fast you are truly on Nature's

operating table without the use of a knife!"

My diseases left my body as a result of fasting. My debts have been discharged. I received invitations to come to different countries and islands. Chapters of this book have unfolded, as well as most of my creative projects and ideas. Fasting has opened space for new possibilities to occur. It has attracted people and resources into my universe.

• Sensual Awakening

As the yogis say, fasting is about holding the senses within, and as a result, they get sharpened. Every time I fast my senses become more acute; I hear better, I can smell better, and my taste buds are more sensitive. My sense of touch is more refined and my skin is smooth and fragrant. My instincts become sharper, and my intuition is unerring.

Fasting is not for everyone. It's a bit like extreme sports. It is for the ones who choose to dare greatly. It's for those who want to champion their life, have amazing sex, and more possibilities. It is an adventure with your body that resets the buttons on everything in your life, including the way you are in bed.

If you are a woman, fasting is going to make you juicy, and boost your appetite for life. It is going to shift your menstruation cycle; the more you fast, the longer your cycle is going to be. You might menstruate as rarely as every 45 days, as opposed to every 28 days. Don't get freaked out. It's normal. That means you will stay young and fertile longer! The same way, you can prepare your body for pregnancy, by fasting before you conceive. You can fast and shed your baby-weight after pregnancy (when you finish nursing).

Fasting will be rejuvenating for you if you are going through menopause and stabilizing your hormones.

If you are a man, fasting will greatly support your fitness, and make you feel like you are 20 years old again. Speaking of the subject that interests you most – i.e. sexuality, you basically last forever. You will become more sensual, more sensitive, and totally in charge of sexual energy, rather than it being in charge of you.

Sound like fun?

My friend Anthony, who is a fasting athlete, long distance runner, and a Gerson therapist, who works with terminally ill patients, speaks honestly about men's health and vitality:

"Once the body of a man is cleansed, the body becomes more aware and sensitive to the internal and external environment. This clean body can connect to another body in an unobstructed way. When you remove obstacles to your sexual energy, your energy flows better!"

• Boosting Immunity

Fasting purifies and oxygenates the blood. It assists the liver in turning the blood from an acid pH into an alkaline pH.

An alkaline environment in your body is an essential prerequisite for strong immunity and vitality.

When your blood is alkaline, your body is able to buffer all sorts of viruses, bacteria, fungi, and parasites, as well as all the thoughts, feelings, and emotions of other people that would otherwise drag you down into a state of stress and dis-ease. Fasting is shedding everything that is not you, whether it is parasites or the energy of other people that act like parasites. Fasting removes all the toxic invaders seeking to colonize your body. As a result, you will be able to reclaim your body, and your life. In short, alkalize or die.

The Western medicine model is erroneously based upon the 19th century germ theory of Louis Pasteur. This French chemist and microbiologist introduced the belief that evil bacteria and viruses attack human bodies for no reason.

Western medical science wants you to believe you are a victim. It wants you to believe illness just all of a sudden happens to you, and there is very little you can do about it, besides taking drugs.

Well, really?

At the same time, when Louis Pasteur put forward his germ theory, another researcher, Antoine Béchamp, was proposing something exactly the opposite. According to him, it was the body's internal condition that was inviting those dangerous microbes to proliferate, multiply and overtake the human body— decomposing it as if it was already dead.

Béchamp was a scientist, while apothecary Pasteur was a chemist with no education in life sciences, and an advertiser, who plagiarized the research of Béchamp, distorted it, and submitted it to the French Academy of Science as his own!

Investigative health reporter Mike Adams, aka Health Ranger, founder of popular web-portal NaturalNews.com, cleared up the confusion between the two theories:

"Pasteur essentially dug up the germ theory of disease and put his name on it." It wasn't a new idea. The concept, which theorizes that many diseases are caused by germs, had actually been outlined by other people many years before. Pasteur nevertheless claimed to have "discovered" germs. Béchamp, on the other hand, proved through original research that most diseases are the result of diseased tissue, and that bacteria and viruses are largely after-effects instead of [the] causes of disease.

Antoine Béchamp was able to scientifically prove that germs are the chemical by-products and constituents of pleomorphic microorganisms enacting upon the unbalanced, malfunctioning cell metabolism and dead tissue that actually produces disease.

Béchamp found that the diseased, acidic, low-oxygen cellular environment is created by a toxic and nutrient-deficient diet, toxic emotions, and a toxic lifestyle. His findings demonstrate how cancer develops through the morbid changes of germs to bacteria, bacteria to viruses, viruses to fungal forms and fungal forms to cancer cells.

After some initial controversy, Pasteur's germ theory ended up winning the day with mainstream medicine—owing in large part to the fact that the theory enabled mainstream medicine to hugely profit from the patented drugs and treatments for fighting germs.

After all, had Béchamp's discoveries been incorporated into current medical curriculum, it would likely have meant a virtual elimination of disease and the end of the pharmaceutical industry."

Béchamp did not believe that bacteria could invade a healthy host and create disease on their own. Instead, he believed that the biological terrain of the being is the cause of disease, not the germ itself. Béchamp claimed that germs and parasites will only survive in acidic and unfavorable conditions, and therefore mere exposure to germs is not enough to get sick.

Béchamp stated, "The primary cause of disease is in us, always in us." Germs and parasites are a little bit like rats that come out on the streets of the cities, where cleaning and maintenance are not observed. It's not the fault of rats, is it? They are just finding food everywhere. In the same way, germs are finding feeding material wherever our blood is acidic, fermenting and where the supply of oxygen is blocked.

Béchamp suggested keeping the body fluids in a high alkaline condition, so that microbes would not be able to breed in it. Pasteur had a devoted following—people acclaiming him a scientific genius.

Pasteur's competing vision became widely accepted by scientists and Béchamp's theories sank into obscurity.

Result? Read Prof. Arnold Ehret's 'Mucusless Diet Healing System. Scientific Method of Eating Your Way To Health':

Since man degenerated thru civilization, he no longer knows what to do when he becomes sick. Disease remains the same mystery to modern medical science as it was to the "Medicine Man" of thousands of years ago - the main difference being that the "germ" theory has replaced the "Demon" and that mysterious outside power still remains - to harm you and destroy life.

A small fringe of dedicated advocates has continued to raise awareness and labor to lead humanity out of the pseudo-scientific superstition. I am certainly one of them. I am here to tell you: There is nothing out there, outside of us, to fear. Nothing can and will penetrate the human body unless we attract it and invite it in by our filthy, unhygienic, acidic lifestyle. This puts the responsibility for your health square on your lap. What you put into your mouth is going to determine whether you compromise your immune system or fortify it. Fasting, cleansing, as well as the raw vegan lifestyle are some of the ways of reclaiming your bioterrain and boosting your own immune system.

It's all about restoring sovereignty in your body. It's also what animals do when they are sick. They fast. Ever since I fasted for the first time in January 2000, I have been able to prevent disease naturally or cure it through natural means, without the need to enter a pharmacy or consult a doctor.

In the words of my favorite Professor again (Arnold Ehret): "...fasting is so feared and misrepresented that the average man actually considers you fool if you miss a few meals when sick, thinking you will starve to death when in reality you are being cured. He fails to understand the difference between fasting and starvation.

Have you ever thought what the lack of appetite means when sick? And that animals have no doctors, and no drug stores, and no sanitariums, and no machinery to heal them? Nature demonstrates and teaches by that example that there is only on disease and that one is cause thru eating - and therefore, every disease whatsoever it may be named by man, is and can be healed by one 'remedy' only - by doing the direct opposite of the cause - by compensation of the wrong - i.e. reducing the quantity of food or fasting."

Rite of Passage

Fasting is more than just non-eating. It is a rite of passage, a farewell to the Old You, and a conscious creation of the New You, the Real You. While you are still in the "passage", it feels like walking through a dark tunnel, with no idea where it's leading you, and what the out-come is going to be. It is all about the art of surrender. Stop everything. Turn off your phone, and your computer. Go within. Your body will tunes in to heal. You won't be able to resist it. There is nothing else to do. Your healing becomes a very beautiful time, indeed. A luxury time when you retreat within you.

Your daily routine is the same. You rise before sunrise, have a coffee enema, make your juice, or if you are lucky enough to live in the tropics, drink coconut water; do yoga, meditate, go for a walk and reflect on your life. When you return, you will drink more, and have a massage or an energy healing session. Then you will drink more, go for a walk, go for a swim, while reflecting on yourself and your life. When you come back, drink more, take your supplements, reflect on your life, take a salt bath. And go to sleep before 8 p.m.

Easy? It's just Drink, drink, drink. Breathe, breathe, breathe. Nowhere to go. Nothing to do.

Herbs & Supplements

Your body is going to cleanse with ease when you receive support in discharging toxins on a cellular level, and purifying your blood. There is a variety of cleansing herbs and supplements that help make this process easy and smooth. Choose products that are raw, organic and a result of cutting-edge research into clinical nutrition, body detoxification processes, energy medicine, and cellular rejuvenation.

Note: most of these raw, organic products have not been approved by the FDA. Manufacturers in America have a big disclaimer on their labels: "Consult your Physician." Your physician most likely has no clue about those products, as they are not part of your doctor's pharmaceutical curriculum, have not been patented and branded by the industry, and there is very little published scientific re-search that would be sponsored to back them up. What an interesting point of view!

Although helpful, supplements and herbs are not necessary. So please, do not turn your home into a vitamin shop. They can be a great ally in your cleanse, but remember — you can do it without them. Nothing in a bottle grows on a tree!

I personally do not use cleansing supplements at all. 'Don't need it. Don't eat it', says my friend Anthony B. Serna. 'Food is something you cannot live without. If you can live without it, it is not food!'

Why Enemas Are So Cool

I love enemas! Love them!

I have witnessed so many healing benefits of coffee enemas, beetroot enemas, herbal enemas, lemon juice enemas, that I cannot possibly hide it, and keep it taboo!

Yeah, agreed! It is not part of our natural state to stick a tube in the butt and flush our bowels with liquid containing coffee! No wild animal does it. Ever. When feeling weak and sick, wild animals will nibble on some herbs, and often refrain from food. Wild animals fast and heal naturally by fasting. According to Dr. Matthias Rath, wild animals do not get cancer. Isn't it interesting? You won't find wild animals eagerly munching on some cheesy canned kitty food, dehydrated puppy food or the tons of genetically modified corn that is fed to livestock. Chickens in South Africa, buffalo in India, geese in Illinois, as well as elk, deer, raccoons, squirrels, mice, and rats have all been seen avoiding genetically modified organisms (GMOs) when given a choice.

Cancer comes together with being chronically domesticated.

A long time ago we used to be wild. However, now we have evolved to become human. We are often told we are only human, as if this was some kind of a curse, handicap or a side effect of the Original Sin.

We are no longer free beings. We take pride in being civilized, and yet we are dumb enough to eat poison, and allow poison into our food. As George Carlin put it: "We have more degrees but less sense, more knowledge, but less judgment, more experts, yet more problems, more medicine, but less wellness."

"Life is a tragedy of nutrition," stated Prof. Arnold Ehret: "Every disease, no matter what name it is known by Medical Science, is Constipation. A clogging up of the entire pipe system of the human body. Any special symptom is therefore merely an extraordinary local constipation by more accumulated mucus at this particular place. Special accumulation points are the tongue, the stomach and particularly the entire digestive tract. This last is the real and deeper cause of bowel constipation. The average person has as much as ten pounds of uneliminated feces in the bowels continually, poisoning the blood stream and the entire system.

The human mechanism is an elastic pipe system. The diet of civilization is never entirely digested and the resultant waste eliminated. This entire pipe system is slowly constipated, especially at the place of the symptom and the digestive tract. This is the foundation of every disease.

Experts in autopsy state they have found that from 60 to 70 percent of the colons examined have foreign matters such as worms and decades-old feces-stones. The inside of walls of the over-intestines are encrusted by old, hardened feces and resemble in appearance the inside of a filthy stove-pipe.

All diseases have their source in the colon, never perfectly emptied since your birth. Nobody on earth today has an ideally clean body and therefore perfectly clean blood. What Medical Science calls normal health is in fact a pathological condition." Enemas are the counterculture of our society. It is impossible for the body to process all the garbage we have been putting inside, so enemas have been created to assist in the process. They are not for good girls and good boys, Ladies and Gentlemen. It's only for the badass among us. It's only for those who dare to unplug from the system and change it.

We certainly do not come out of our mama's bellies with an enema bag or bucket, but then again we aren't meant to eat all that crap we are eating. David Wolfe, the super-food guru and bestselling author, once put it directly: "We have been eating stuff that should not even be in landfills."

This is especially true of American people who have been incrementally swindled to consume ever-increasing doses of highly addictive pseudo-food substances: MSG, aspartame, corn syrup, hormones, pesticides and the biggest lie of all, the genetically modified organisms. Americans have been drugged beyond measure in their homes, vaccinated at schools, and medicated in hospitals, and are now being prescribed synthetic heroine painkillers by their own family doctors.

If you believe that people will detox their body with ease, just by drinking kale juice every day, taking shots of wheat grass juice, and going vegan, or even fruitarian, you are being naive. The side effects of cleansing can be horrible and unbearable to someone who is coming off the FDA-approved Standard American Diet (SAD, indeed!). Headaches, nausea, diarrhea, and muscle cramps are common. It's very similar to a drug addict coming off his dope. Beware! The road to bliss is not always blissful. It can be tormenting!

This is why enemas make this process so much easier by supporting the body in discharging all the toxins. Thank God we have this technique to help flush toxins more easily. I cannot even imagine fasting without coffee enemas. This practice saved my life, and I am totally grateful to Nadia who taught me to use it.

And heck, if I can do it, so can you!

A coffee enema in the morning lays the foundation for your cleanse during the day. It sets the energy wherein you get back the control over your own body, and reclaim your sovereignty. Coffee enemas soften the walls of the colon and remove the zoo of alien microbes residing in the colon that tend to rule the appetite. These alien microbes send signals to the brain that feel like cravings on your tongue: "We want a steak! We want ice cream! We want pizza!" Do you know why? Because they want to multiply, and they can do so only if your insides ferment, rot, petrify and choke with no oxygen, and slowly die. The problem is that they want to take over while you are still living, because the environment of your body liquids is acidic and very inviting.

And here comes the enema secret:

Don't worry. You are not lazy. You do not have a weak will, so stop blaming yourself every time you reach out for some junk. The system got you addicted, and the parasites inside your colon rule. The time has come to reclaim your body and give parasites the finger!

A coffee enema helps your body to get rid of all the toxic residue, yeast and microbes in the colon... All that zoo that's craving processed food. It assists in releasing gallbladder stones and colon stones, and allows your blood to purify. How does it get any better than that?

During the fast, I have a coffee enema first thing in the morning as I wake up before the sunrise. It clears my mind, calms me down, stops my cravings and gives me energy for the day. Thanks to the morning enema, I can fast the whole day with ease, without craving any solid food.

When people give up and quit cleansing and start eating, I always know they didn't do one thing: the coffee enema first thing in the morning. If they did, they would not crave food. "First thing" means the first thing you do when you wake up at 6 a.m., not later. You should prepare the liquid before you go to sleep, so you have it ready when you get up, and only need to warm it up. Especially since you might wake up feeling a little foggy, weak, and not in the mood to do anything.

During your sleep time, your body will process and release toxins out of your cells, lymph and bloodstream, and bring it all into the colon. When your colon is clogged up, so is your brain. In Chinese medicine, the brain and the colon are very connected. You will feel foggy, tired, and moody. I notice when I am fasting, a coffee enema first thing in the morning clears my brain right away! After the enema I feel increased energy levels, more clarity, and a sense of euphoria.

Coffee is a medicine and it was never meant to be taken orally, as when you drink it from your favorite coffee mug in the office or at the coffee shop.

When you drink coffee, it stimulates your sympathetic nervous system, which is responsible for the wave con-traction of peristalsis in your digestive tract. It will sharpen your brain for a while, but unfortunately it will acidify your blood, and alienate you from your body and your feelings. It will soon give you a highand-low roller coaster.

When coffee is ingested by mouth, it is digested by stomach acids and enzymes, and most of its herbal medicine properties are destroyed.

However, when taken rectally via an enema, the coffee goes directly to the liver through the colon wall, where it stimulates the para-sympathetic system, which is responsible for stimulation of "rest-and-digest" activities, such as urination, digestion and defecation. It also stimulates glutathione production, known as the "mother of all antioxidants".

Coffee is not food, and not a drink; the beans are actually a medicine that has been commercialized into the Western lifestyle. One of its properties is to function as an astringent herb, peeling the top layer of skin or mucous membrane. This is helpful, as the top layer of skin or mucous membrane is often ready to come off anyway, and is loaded with toxins. So it is like cleaning the surface layer of the mucous membrane of the colon and the liver as well.

The editors of Physiological Chemistry and Physics stated "Caffeine enemas cause dilation of bile ducts, which facilitates excretion of toxic cancer breakdown products by the liver and dialysis of toxic products from blood across the colonic wall."

Dr. Max Gerson, MD, the major proponent of the coffee enema in the Western world, wrote that:

"Heubner and Meyer of Goettingen University, Germany, had shown in animal models that rectal administration of caffeine would dilate bile ducts and promote bile flow. The introduction of a quart of coffee solution into the colon will dilute portal blood and subsequently, the bile. Theophylline and theobromine, major constituents of coffee, dilate blood vessels and counter inflammation of the gut. The palmitates of coffee enhance glutathione S-transferase, which is responsible for the removal of many toxic radicals from serum.

Finally, the fluid of the enema itself stimulates the visceral nervous system, promoting peristalsis and the transit of diluted toxic bile from the duodenum out through the rectum.

Because the stimulating enema is retained for 15 minutes, and because all the blood in the body passes through the liver nearly every three minutes, these enemas represent a form of dialysis of the blood across the gut wall."

Here's what Dr. Gabriel Cousens, an outstanding MD and expert on cleansing, writes about enemas in his online article, The Coffee Enema: Its Unique History & Amazing Detox Properties:

"An enema is a fluid injected into the rectum for the purpose of clearing out the bowel, or of administering drugs or food. The word itself comes from the Greek 'enhienai', meaning to send or inject into. The enema has been called one of the oldest medical procedures still used today. Tribal women in Africa, and elsewhere, routinely use it on their children. The earliest medical text in existence, the Egyptian Ebers Papyrus, from 1500 B.C., mentions it.

Millennia before, the Pharaoh had a guardian of the anus, a special doctor, one of whose purposes was to ad-minister the royal enema.

Yogis in India and the ancient Egyptians have used the coffee enema since ancient times. The Greeks wrote of the fabled cleanliness of the Egyptians, which included the internal cleansing of their systems through emetics and enemas. They employed these on three consecutive days a month said Herodotus, or at intervals of three or four days, according to a later historian Diodorus Siculus. The Egyptians explained to their visitors that they did this because they believed that diseases were engendered by superfluities of the food, a modern-sounding theory!

Enemas were known in ancient Sumeria, Babylonia, India, Greece, and China. Native Americans independently invented it, using a syringe made of an animal bladder and a hollow leg bone. Pre-Columbian South Americans fashioned latex into the first rubber enema bags and tubes. In fact, there is hardly a region of the world where people did not discover or adapt the enema. It is more ubiquitous than the wheel. Enemas are found in world literature from Aristophanes to Shakespeare, Gulliver's Travels to Peyton Place.

In pre-revolutionary France, a daily enema after dinner was de rigueur. It was not only considered indispensable for health but also practiced for good complexion as well. Louis XIV is said to have taken over 2,000 in his lifetime. Could this have been the source of the Sun King's sunny disposition? For centuries, enemas were a routine home remedy. In recent times, the routine use of enemas died out. The main circumstances where doctors employ them nowadays are before and after surgery and right before childbirth. Difficult and potentially dangerous barium enemas before colonic X-rays are of course still a favorite among allopathic doctors."

Learning how to do an enema is empowering. It makes you sovereign, and you do not need to depend on anyone else. It nurtures independence and builds a relationship with your body like nothing else. In addition to a coffee enema, you can have a chlorophyll or herbal enema, raw beet juice enema, hydrogen peroxide enema or an enema with fulvic acid, etc. These options are not always available when you have colonics. On the other hand, colonic hydrotherapy will flush and hydrate your intestines thoroughly, something I do at least twice a year.

Enemas or colonics are the best-kept secret of many celebrities in the showbiz industry. Lady Diana kept her radiant beauty with regular colonics and enemas. Many of my celebrity clients do the same to rejuvenate and stay young, although they won't tell you their secret on TV. If they did, their agent would call the next day with a warning that they will not get any more roles in movies and commercials. It's gross, after all! For some reason, main-stream media conditions the Western Woman to throw on a ton of make-up, wear the latest high-heels, and carry the latest designer's handbag, while at the same time she rots inside.

That's not considered gross, but a hygiene procedure that would help her to cleanse and rejuvenate from inside out is taboo. It's considered disgusting. Is it because she would become a dangerously gorgeous natural female? Is it because her skin would be smooth, fragrant and glowing and she wouldn't need to hide behind the makeover lie? Or is it because she would be healthy?

Quoting Prof. Arnold Ehret again: "On the outside, the man of today is carefully groomed, perhaps unnecessarily and over carefully clean; while inside he is dirtier than the dirtiest animal - whose anus is as clean as its mouth, provided said animal has not been 'domesticated' by 'civilized' man."

Well, if we got healthy, Ladies and Gentlemen, someone would lose a lot of money.

No wonder colonic hydrotherapy was systematically removed from American hospitals during World War II, exactly when Rockefeller's and JP Morgan's "business with disease" model was systematically introduced.

Today, it consists of pharmaceutical cartels that sponsor all the pseudo-scientific research. Given the healing benefits of coffee enemas, no wonder there is no research on the topic. There is little besides the pharma-sponsored disinformation campaign on the Internet. Most medical doctors will not recommend an enema. They never had one!

In Ukraine, an enema bag is not taboo. I've seen it hanging in the bathroom. When I asked my host about it, the answer was simple:

"We cannot afford to get sick. We do not have money to go to a hospital."

That's the way you think when you don't have insurance and you need to be smart and take care of yourself. Have you noticed? People who do not have insurance recover faster than those who do? Does it make you wonder why? Remember, as long as someone else takes care of you, you do not take care of yourself! Learning how to give yourself coffee enemas is the first step to your own path of "Know thyself. Heal thyself ".

Dr. Gabriel Cousens continues:

"Dr. Max Gerson used coffee enemas clinically as part of a general detoxification regimen, first for tuberculosis, then cancer. Caffeine, he postulated, will travel up the hemorrhoidal [vein] to the portal vein and then to the liver. Gerson noted some remarkable effects of this procedure. For instance, patients did not need their usually prescribed painkillers once on the enemas. Many people have noted the paradoxical calming effect of coffee enemas. And while coffee enemas can relieve constipation,

Gerson cautioned: 'Patients have to know that the coffee enemas are not given for the function of the intestines but for the stimulation of the liver'.

Coffee enemas were an established part of medical practice when Dr. Max Gerson introduced them into cancer therapy in the 1930s. Basing himself on German laboratory work, Gerson believed that caffeine could stimulate the liver and gallbladder to discharge bile. He felt this process could contribute to the health of the cancer patient."

Today, coffee enemas are part of the basic ABCs you will learn at the renowned Gerson Institute Clinics (one in Hungary and one in Mexico), where cancer patients flock from all over the world. The therapy is so effective that it actually has been officially banned from American hospitals.

OK. Here's how I do it!

It is much easier to film it than to describe it with words. Though, if I filmed it, I would probably become an X-rated Super Star! (Well, now you got me thinking!)

I boil purified water in a huge 2-gallon pot. In a 2-quart saucepan I boil ground organic coffee and simmer it for 10 minutes. Green coffee is slightly roasted and is better for an enema. Dark coffee is just as good if I do not have access to green coffee. It is exactly the same coffee I would use to make espresso, except that when I use dark coffee, I boil it and let it simmer for 10-15 minutes, then strain it and pour it into the big pot of clear water, thus turning the water into a slightly brown color.

I make sure my coffee enema water in the big pot is warm before I take it to the bathroom. I pour the liquid into my enema bucket (some use an enema bag, but a bucket is much easier). That means that I might need to wait for it to cool down. If I prepare it the night before, I warm it in the morning. I always check with my finger to ensure the temperature is lukewarm. It should not be hot or cold. It should be lukewarm, to match the temperature inside my colon.

There are many enema kits out there on the market. They vary in sizes, prices, and models. An enema kit consists of either a bucket or a 2 or 4-quart rubber latex bag, and tubing that connects the bag to the nozzle, which will be inserted into the rectum.

An ideal kit uses a stainless steel bucket, as the large capacity eliminates refilling during the enema. The container should be easy to clean and must not "age" with use. Enema bags suffer on both counts. They cannot be cleaned effectively and often the latex "sweats" over time. Containers of stainless steel are preferable.

The enema tubing (hose) should preferably be latex-free and transparent, which allows you to see the fluid flow during the enema. There should also be an adjustable "pinch" clamp over the tubing to easily manage liquid flow. The colon tube or enema insertion tip should preferably be sterilized and replaceable as well as latex-free.

Silicone is a great material for enema equipment because it is nonporous, hypoallergenic and can be disinfected easily. I like to use a stainless steel enema bucket, since it is solid and I can set it on the bathroom counter and pour the coffee water into it.

If you are on a limited budget you might opt for a simple latex 2-quart enema bag that will also serve as a hot water bottle. Make sure it comes with that option.

I take the large 2-gallon pot with coffee water into the bathroom, and place it on the floor. I place the enema kit at the sink level or higher so the water can flow down by gravity. If using an enema bag, you can simply hang it on a towel hook or a shower curtain rod, etc. I lubricate the nozzle (colon tip) with coconut oil, or olive oil. I pour the liquid inside the container, while having the hose clamp closed.

I spread an old beach towel on the floor and kneel down "doggy style" (smile), and insert the lubricated tube into the rectum. I open the clamp and allow the liquid to flow. I close the clamp when I feel I have enough liquid in my body, and can't take in any more. I swoosh it around in my belly, jump, dance, and massage my abdomen to make the most of it, and this hydrates the colon even more to unglue the fecal matter from its walls, and besides it adds a bit of fun. Aha! When I can't hold it in any more, I sit on the toilet, and Niagara Falls!

If I have a little stool handy, I like to put my feet on it, to get close to a squatting position while sitting on the toilet. Guess what? That's how we used to poop, before the toilet was invented, and that odd squatting position gets all the poop out of the colon at once. This squatting position causes the puborectalis muscle to fully relax, allowing the colon to open and empty quickly and completely.

When done, I keep going ahead with the next round until the entire 2-gallon pot is empty. I may change positions during this process to thoroughly hydrate the colon. I can lie down with my back on the towel and put my feet up. I can roll over onto the right side to make sure the water will get into my entire intestine, and this helps to flush out the liver stones.

At the beginning, I was lucky if I got to keep the water inside for more than a minute. With most people, the colon lining is hardened by the toxins that are sticking onto the wall and the colon stones that have formed over years have deformed the shape of the colon itself. Coffee water softens the intestinal lining and helps to discharge it. So don't worry if you just take the water in and feel like going back on the toilet seat immediately. Bravo! Keep doing that, and you will be surprised how your belly will go down, while your colon will be able to receive and hold more and more of the liquid.

How To Forgive Radically

I have yet to meet anyone healthy who has not forgiven. Here's how you can forgive radically!

And—how do you know you have forgiven?

You are Grateful!

I meet many people diagnosed with cancer and I always ask them what happened in their life just before it was discovered. Some are surprised why I dare to ask. It brings up painful memories.

I have noticed that always there is some kind of trauma, some kind of a shock to the system, some kind of an event that caused sadness, stress, resentment, guilt, blame, or shame. Sometimes, this depressive condition continues for a chronic period of time before the illness is discovered. Sometimes, it is very short and sudden.

It all centers on one thing: Judgment.

Always, some kind of judgment has been passed out that caused an avalanche of overwhelming thoughts, feelings and emotions that literally swamped the body with acid. From experience, I have discovered there is nothing more acidic than judgment.

Life is not all roses. Life has many surprises. Many situations happen that are facts. They really did take place. However, it is up to us to create drama-loaded judgment over the facts, or simply see them for what they are. Even when it comes to subjects as sensitive as sexual abuse, it still is what it is. How you interpret the event will either empower you or destroy you. You can look at the event as a fact – it happened, and say to yourself: 'So What?' Or you can create a story and decide you are now broken forever.

Your body records the memory of everything you experience. All your thoughts, feelings and emotions, judgments, decisions, conclusions and computations have been recorded in your body. What if 98% of it is not even yours? Who does it belong to? Would you like to shed that weight?

These memories are stored in your cellular membrane. According to Bruce H. Lipton, Ph.D., our cells bathe in the energy and vibration created by our thoughts.

Dr. Lipton, an internationally recognized cellular biologist and a pioneer in the new science of epigenetics (epi: *above*; genetics: *origins*—the study of the role of experiences and emotions upon our bodies and health) argues scientifically that it is not our genes that create illness, it is our mind. If the mind is sick, there is no way for the body to be healthy!

Attention! This makes you the creator of your disease, right? Yes. It takes you out of the notion of being a victim. A dangerous idea! If you have created disease, what else can you create? What if you can create bliss??

Chinese medicine, and other ethnic healing systems of the world, also contends that our body organs store emotions. For example, the liver stores anger, the kidneys store fear, the spleen retains worries, the lungs hold onto sadness, and the colon is a repository for all sorts of unconscious, repressed emotions of which we are not even aware. Best proof? When people have organ transplants, they feel emotions and inherit memories from the donor!

Do not just take my word for it. Cleanse your body and you will see for yourself how you will not be able to get angry, or hold on to a grudge, or feel sadness, or buy into other people's drama. You will feel your own energy and you will be in charge.

When you forgive you reset your body's computer and discharge all those negative, redundant memories, all those broken records. This is why I recommend practicing Radical Forgiveness.

Radical Forgiveness is a profound healing technique described by Colin Tipping in his groundbreaking book under the same title.

Before you do it, go into a state of meditation, and create harmonious ambiance around you. Call upon your angels, ancestors, Mother Earth, Mother Mary, whoever or whatever you believe is working with you. You are going to clear your 'karma' now. You are inviting them to witness.

Get paper and pen. You are going to write three letters. Do not stop until you finish writing. Pour it all out on pa-per without judgment, without censorship, or editing. Cry if you need to.

No one is going to read these letters. They are for you to express all the thoughts, feelings and emotions that are not even yours and have been in your body for a long time. You are going to date, sign and burn them when you finish writing.

Visualize in front of you the person that you believe hurt you, and write. Do not judge what you have written, just write. Pour all the thoughts, feelings and emotions out on the paper until you empty yourself. Do not stop writing until you are done. Consider that what happened in your life is a fact. However, your judgment of the situation—right or wrong, good or bad—is a story.

Who would you be without your story? What's left after you shed all the judgments? Just You, and the greatness of You!

Go ahead. Write.

Letter No. 1: Emotional Purging

The first letter is an emotional release of all the build up of anger, sadness, and disappointment. Write the story of how you've been hurt, abused, mistreated, etc. If you feel like cursing, go ahead. Pour it all out. Don't send this letter, okay? When you are done, sign it, date it, and burn it. This is a clearing for your emotional body. It is a way you can detoxify your cellular memory.

Letter No. 2: Psychological Forgiveness

In this letter you come up with all the rational excuses for the person's behavior that hurt you: "I know you couldn't act differently, because you were abused when you were a child, etc. I forgive you."

It's the way we have been taught to forgive in this reality. Does it really help you to forget? It doesn't. Do it any-way. This letter is meant for your mind to understand why something happened. It is all about looking at things from another perspective.

Letter No. 3: Soul-to-Soul Forgiveness

The third letter is magic. If you write the first two letters with depth, the third one is going to bring you relief, joy and gratitude. You don't have to believe it, just write:

"I remember before we incarnated here on Earth, we met in the spirit planes where we designed our future lives on this planet. I have chosen a certain mission here on Earth. I needed someone to come and give me suffering so that I would learn fast and grow. Your soul has volunteered to make a sacrifice for me and has stepped in as my teacher to accelerate my learning. You appeared in a dark, manipulative energy of an aggressor, and I believed you. You played a role in my life that helped me grow. I acknowledge that it must have been so difficult for your soul to be in that energy. I honor your sacrifice. I am so grateful. I promise you from now on that I will be more joyful than ever, more powerful, more vigilant, more creative and happier than ever!"

You can even choose a project you'd like to accomplish in honor of your teacher-in-disguise.

How do you know you have forgiven? When you are grateful!

Sometimes, those letters of Radical Forgiveness take more than one day. That's great! I continue to fast as I write them! If you write those letters, and you are not in tears, you are probably not writing them deeply enough. Most likely you are not allowing yourself to remember how deeply you were hurt. You need to know what you are forgiving, look at your pain, and watch the scary movie to the end, before your insane mind is ready to let go.

Radical Forgiveness will allow you to empty yourself of all the guilt-blame-and-shame games. As you detoxify on a physical level by fasting, you also detoxify on an emotional, intellectual, and energetic level through Radical Forgiveness.

This process will bring you joy, gratitude and lightness. This letting go of the emotional cause of acidity is a precondition for your blood to be alkaline. Toxic emotions make our blood acidic. Wanna be healthy? Forgive Radically!

Some say we need to come to God empty-handed. If we still hold grudges, the angels look and say: "Oh, you are still holding grudges. Please come back when your hands are empty! We will give you some goodies!" and they do! Abundance is awaiting those who forgive. If you are stuck in your financial life somewhere, fast and forgive. It will open you to receive.

Buddha said: "Failing to forgive is like drinking poison and hoping someone else will get sick." It doesn't work that way, does it? If you drink the poison of toxic thoughts, feelings, and emotions, it is really your blood that you poison!

At the same time, the one you hold the grudge against might be oblivious of the situation. Yes! They may be insensitive, or very dense, or blocked, and therefore unaware and didn't notice that they ever hurt you!

A client I have worked with in the past was raped by her hypnotherapist. She gained weight to protect herself from men. She did not want to forgive and let go of the past. She was resistant to writing these letters. Despite the coconut water fast, and herbs, and enemas, she was not losing weight. Not even a pound!

I recommended that she stay at home and write the letters of Radical Forgiveness until she finished, instead of going with us to the beach. She kept writing the entire day, and cried, facing her memories. Finally, she wrote the third letter, and cried with tears of gratitude while burning it. In the night, she woke up several times with diarrhea and vomiting. Her body shed three pounds in just that one night.

How about you? Whose weight are you carrying? Who does it belong to? Who do you need to forgive? Is now the time to be authentic and honest about it?

In Landmark Forum, where forgiveness is key in healing relationships, the forum leader encourages the participant to make a phone call immediately to the person they are in a relationship with and actually admit they've been unauthentic, pretending and dishonest, what it cost them, what has been missing for them both, and what's possible now. The process is extremely powerful, restores integrity, and brings freedom.

Sacred Time

Fasting is a sacred time for you – for your body and your spirit. It is not the time to drive around town and do errands. It is not the time to watch TV, carry on phone conversations, do business or keep texting with friends.

Your cleanse is the unique time you can allocate to purify your body and to reflect upon your life. Yes. You might not feel comfortable with what you will find out, however, you might be empowered on a cellular level to change your life—from the core of your being, from the inside out.

Going through a cleanse purely on a physical level neglects this important aspect of your being. It might result in an emotional crisis, and cause emotional outbursts. For this reason, Radical Forgiveness is a tool for cleansing the mind as you cleanse your body.

The Native Hawaiian Kahunas (highly respected healers and community leaders) are very big on forgiveness. They call it Ho'oponopono, which means to make right. One Kahuna I met stated: "If you are sick, whom do you need to forgive? If you are in financial struggle, whom do you need to forgive?"

Forgive and you will feel as light as a feather. If you seek Enlightenment, here's your first step. Forgive and take things lightly from now on.

Cancer is always proceeded by an event, some kind of a deep, overwhelming tragedy that caused hurt, pain and suffering. Most often, the event occurred first time in childhood and what's happening now is just an echo of the trauma. The story can be different from person to person. The energy always feels the same. It doesn't let us sleep through the night.

Interestingly enough, all women with ovarian cancer that I ever met and interviewed, have been sexually molested in childhood. I know I was, and I know self-healing processes, such a Radical Forgiveness and Landmark Forum, have helped me to transform this pain into a profound source of strength, freedom and liberation. Today, I don't know how would I be able to lead and empower, if I did not go through it, and if I did not transmute this copper into gold.

"I wrote my Radical Forgiveness Letters,' says Jessica R., from Los Angeles who's been on cleansing and healing from ovarian cancer. 'For the first time I've been able to sleep through the night. I feel great. I feel I am going to succeed.'

Sylvia Ray Arden, the singer-song writer who has graced this book with her personal foreword, has undergone a profound inner healing journey to overcome her ovarian cancer. Here's her account of the process:

"One of the most essential parts of my healing from ovarian cancer, was the emotional and spiritual Rite of Passage. The trauma healing, meeting and recovering the inner child, the rebirth of the True Self.

It has been a residual energy from years and decades of abusive childhood and although I was not quite ready yet to take a look at this part prior to my diagnosis, this time there was no easier or softer way through it, there was no more running away from myself and from Life.

The time has come for me to take a deeper look, to dive in and surrender to whatever was on the way to be revealed at the level of my pain body, as Eckhart Tolle might have brilliantly said in his book 'the Power of Now'.

I has been extremely painful to confront the abuse and the trauma yet once again, but as I was facing death, the question was: Was I really able to run away again? Was I about to hide and freeze my emotions and feelings once again in order to survive? The old methods of fight, flight and fright syndrome, seem not to have work this time.

And I truly was so fed up with my Life's experiences, that it was not about surviving and running away any longer.The time has come to decide: either to live fully, to thrive, or die.

The Divine Guidance, Spirit, the so called Higher Power, was calling me to heal profoundly and this time I have found enough trust within, safety, guidance and willingness to do so.

I remember, in the second month of my healing journey, in the middle of the night, as I was lying in bed praying for a miracle and the trees and winds were announcing, that there was something about to emerge, a whispering, yet powerful call for change. I was wide awake.

It was 2 am.. I couldn't sleep...I was crying, tears were flowing down my face as if on autopilot. I felt a pounding abdominal pain in the area where the tumor was located, on the left side, my female side, in the Realm of the Moon Goddess Reign.

It was there, a peaceful yet assertive voice was proclaiming: "You have to take a look at one of the most terrifying and devastating experiences of your Life: the sexual abuse and the trauma."

So I did.

I saw a sweet, little, innocent, precious, beautiful little girl, my inner child, all alone in the darkness, petrified and scared to death. She was in tremendous pain, indescribable terror and so very alone and deeply sad. It was me calling for help, me asking the grown up woman, to take care of myself, to love myself, cherish and finally liberate myself.

I was deeply moved, the vision and the process was so real as the fact that I was there lying in bed, weeping in the middle of the night..

My heart was wide open, yet tearing apart from the horrifying pain I have felt.

I was 'shouting' within: HOW could all this be possible? All the rapes, all the violence, all these horrific experiences that definitely do not belong to the treasured and fragile time of being a child and growing up. Well no! These type of experiences do NOT belong in anybody's Life. NO one's Life and I mean NOONE's... NOBODY, neither male or female... NO! PERIOD...

FINITO... NO!

I felt so damn angry, I felt a rage building up inside like an avalanche taking over the mountain .. pacing down the sculptures of the earth.

I felt a cleansing fire in my Solar Plexus area, like the Sycamore Tree fires burning down what's no longer working, what is done and gone, outdated, toxic, the injustice and the insanity, that what wasn't even mine in the first place. The world the Patriarchy and the Hierarchy... Who made these rules? I am so confused. Well, certainly not me. The cleansing fires of the Sycamore tree; the death of the old in order for the new to arise.

I suddenly saw myself as my own loving, nurturing mother, with an overwhelming feeling of gentleness, kindness, wisdom, compassion and care for my own little girl. I literally felt, as I visualized, embracing myself, hugging myself so lovingly and deeply, gently, proclaiming: ' I am here right here my Love, you no longer have to go through this, I am picking you up and taking you with me my Love,.my most precious Love...You are being taking care of deeply, profoundly, you are safe now.. you are the most beautiful and talented little girl in the world and you deserve the best in Life..

Somehow, Louise L Hay's words of wisdom, were ringing a bell suddenly. All that I have ever learned, the countless affirmations I was practicing, the metaphysical laws, quantum physics, law of attraction and law of polarity, everything that I was studying and pursuing over the years of hardship and up's and down's, trial and error, was finally making a greater sense.. Better yet, I felt it deep in my Heart and Soul and Spirit. I was finally downloading it, assimilating... All the wisdom, all the knowledge. All the authentic, true precious Self. What a gift.

What a blessing. The real meaning behind the words, or as Evita would say: *The Bliss of Cancer...*

And as intense and intimate this experience has been, on the physical level, I felt my cancer tumor was buzzing, tingling. I felt a symbiosis of pleasure and pain, a profound healing was taking place.

Conscious and subconscious transformation, a transition from darkness to light, from hell to heaven.

I cannot emphasize and stress enough, how imperative the spiritual and emotional part of the healing process is, in order to overcome any kind of disease or so called dysfunction in the body.

I encourage everyone to dive deep within and look for the treasures hidden on the intangible sides of our existence. To go through the angst of the rite of passage in order to heal, is a gift in estrange wrapping paper, as on the other side of the tunnel is the light, the bliss, the freedom and the divine love that we came to this existence with, in the first place."

Why Fat Is So Bad

No wild animals eat fat. And they do not have cancer...

You read at the beginning of this book that I did something very weird in order to heal myself. I had to drink a disgusting concoction of extra virgin olive oil and grapefruit juice. People call this procedure 'liver flush'. The idea behind is that drinking large quantity of oil shocks the liver and forces it to release gallbladder stones. Well... I have news for you. You do not have to do that. Today, knowing what I know about health and wellness, I know it was Granny Smith apple juice that healed me, and my decision to own my life. Not oil. Today, I would never do that again, or recommend that you would have to do it.

Especially, if someone has cancer and their body organs are weak, last thing they should do is to drink oil. It may cause bloating, and – worst thing – we don't know how long does the oil stay in the body before it is discharged. We have no idea. Andreas Moritz, the man who advocated this treatment, died at the age of 58. Kind of young, don't you think?

I discovered a different path of healing. It leads through yumminess, bliss and delight. And there is nothing yummy about drinking oil or eating fat.

Human being is the only 'animal' that will eat butter, or butter-like avocados. Domesticated animals will eat virtually everything humans will give them, which is why they are coming up with cancers and other 'civilized diseases'. We humans lose instincts in domestication, and out common sense is no longer common!

"Don't you know that bookbinder's paste is made of white flour, rice or potatoes?", asks prof. Arnold Ehret. "That glue is made from flesh gristle and bones? Don't know how sticky these substances are? Don't you know that skimmed milk, buttermilk and cream are the best ingredients used to furnish a sticky base for color for painting? That the white of eggs will stick paper or cloths so perfectly that it resists dissolution in water? Every housewife and cook knows how oils and fats stick to the sides of a pan. At least 90 per cent of the "diet of civilization" contains these sticky foods and man stuffs himself daily with awful mixtures of them. Thus the digestive tract is not only clogged up through constipation, but literally glued together with sticky mucus and feces."

Let's ask then what would we eat, if we were free – from birth, uncultured, uncivilized...

Imagine you never went to school. Imagine you didn't even grow up in a human home. (Maybe the wolves raised you, Mowgli?!) You weren't spoon-fed by your Mama. Daddy didn't blackmail you at the dining table: 'Hey! You better clear your plate, if you want to watch the cartoons tonight'. There was no Christmas candy cane, no school canteen, no drive in restaurants, or dinner parties. You have no idea what humans eat. You just arrived here.

You walk in the mountains, in wilderness, and you need to survive. What are you going to do? You are really hungry. Are you going to kill a cow that's feeding on the meadow? Are you salivating when you look at it? Are you feeling like peeling off the skin and biting into the raw flesh? Not really. It's a big project. You require tools and some help. Maybe two of you, or three to carry the pray... That's a lot of effort.

You are hungry now. Right now!

Are you going to try to catch a bird? Do you salivate when you look at it? Do you feel like plucking the feathers, biting into the flesh? Not really, ha?

How about fish? Do you salivate when you look at fish swimming in the creek? Are you going to jump in and try to catch it? You obviously don't have time to make a fishing rod. You are hungry now!

What will satisfy that hunger within you now - right now? What would be the quickest, easiest to obtain food around you? The easiest to pick? The easiest to put apart? What do you salivate for?

Nuts! You think? You look at macadamia tree. You pick one nut and try to crack it. Not easy! Rewarding on the inside however. You try to crack the next one. That one didn't turn out so yummy, and was so hard to open. It was rancid inside. You try another one. This one is better, but you are tried of it. Lots of work and not much food.

You gravitate towards fruit – for the colors seduce you. The texture, the symmetry, the sunshine glittering inside when you bite in. You salivate when you look at it, and even more when you smell it. Touching a peach gives you pleasure. Looking at grapes reminds you of paradise... And – they are so easy to obtain. Apples fall off the trees when you rest in the shade. Berries are almost begging to be picked. Bananas, oranges, mangos, papayas are in every jungle you roam.

Avocados? Lots of them. They grow on trees, and many already fell on the ground. The colors do not look too appealing, neither does the texture. You bite into one. Interesting. Soft and buttery. You have another bite, and another, and yet another; and you begin to choke. There is something missing there. There is no juice, no oxygen... You realize, it's not something that can sustain you. It is not something you can feed on every day, the whole day, several times a day. In other words, it's not your food.

Oil? It never occurs in nature.

That fairytale basically tells the story. The story of the Garden of Eden we once used to live in, and we need to return to if we want to heal. Humans have gone so far from the paradise paradigm that they are addicted to fat, and - though it kills them in sophisticated ways - many will die to defend it.

And, yes! There are two kinds of fat: animal fat and plantbased fat. I will surprise you by saying it doesn't matter! Fat is fat. It has a similar density, structure, and no amount of water in it. It is what parasites crave inside us - in order to breed.

Prof. Arnold Ehret taught his students: "All fats are acid forming, even those of vegetable origin, and are not used by the body. You will continue to like, crave and use them only as long as you can still see mucus in the 'magic mirror' (white coating on your tongue). What doctors call heat calories is caused by the fats in friction, obstruction in the circulation; they constipate the small blood vessels."

He knew this truth will be a hard sell: "No scientific food value tables can convince you of the truth. You must sense it with your cleansed organs, how wrongly you are fooled into believing that you nourish and build up health and efficiency by these foods which are in reality destructive, because they stimulate, or more truthfully, stop the elimination of your old waste until the day of reckoning comes, when you become 'officially' sick."

There is an abundance of scientific research and evidence on the benefits of olive oil, flaxseed oil, or coconut oil. There is a million blog posts written on the healing power of raw soaked almonds, nut milk or avocado. Please do not think, I am not familiar with any of it. The quantity recommended varies from one school of nutrition to another, from one naturopath to the other, from one health guru's bible to another one's.

However, I do not go by science, or by a book. I listen to my own body. Ever since I healed, my body is pure and it speaks to me. It gives me feedback. If I eat something good for me – I have lots of energy. I feel light, and inspired. If I eat something toxic, I feel constipated, sleepy, tired, bloated, foggy, moody, and I get pimples.

No amount of science is going to fool it. The body never lies.

Try this experiment. Slice a strawberry and prepare it to be a rejuvenating strawberry facial mask. Fabulous! So many vitamins for your skin! Now, do something crazy. Put olive oil, coconut oil, or apply avocado on your face. Spread it evenly. And now – try putting the strawberry mask on your skin. Is it going to do any good? Not at all! Why is that? Because the pores of your skin are all clogged up by the fat, right? Now, envision. The same is happening in the body, except it's amplified by internal heat. The temperature inside your digestive tract is way higher than on your cheeks. The fat you consume becomes rancid very quickly and our strawberry goes into fermentation.

I have been watching my own body, and receiving feedback from many people I work with. Here's my observation on what fat does to the body:

Fat causes cancer.

Fat blocks oxygen supply. Fat clogs up tissues, arteries, digestive tract and blocks oxygen. Cancer thrives in an environment that lacks oxygen. It is a fantastic environment for parasites. The body is choking internally, while fat goes rancid inside causing fermentation of fruit and decay of protein. The clogged up tissues are not able to absorb the vital nutrients that come from fruits and vegetables, or juices. These just go in and out – at best – or stay inside blocked in the colon and becoming a food for candida. The body is malnourished, and its immune system becomes compromised. Tumors form in areas that are most clogged up.

Fat causes candida overgrowth.

Candida normally is our ally. It eats up the surplus of sugar that would otherwise ferment inside the colon. However, when colon is clogged up by fat on the walls, fruit doesn't get absorbed and candida just has too much food. It breeds more than normal. It's not caused by fruit though. Fruit normally gets absorbed within seconds and there is not much left for candida to breed. Fat blocks absorption and causes candida overgrowth.

Fat causes heart-disease

Fat accumulates around the veins and clogs them up. As a result they become more narrow and the blood pressure increases. See the footage from any heart surgery!

Fat causes diabetes

Fat blocks insulin supply, and clogs up micro-veins and capillaries thus diminishing blood flow into extremities. It leads to numbing of fingers and hands, or amputation of limbs.

Fat causes sexual diseases

Fat makes blood acidic, overloaded with mucus and pus. The body in this condition becomes prone to all sorts of infections and viruses that would otherwise never set in. It causes urinary track infections, bladder infections, vaginal dryness, menstruation pain, menopause hot flashes, hormonal imbalance, sexual impotency, etc.

Fat causes depression and mental disorders.

Fat blocks oxygen in the body. Without oxygen, it is impossible to be happy and think clearly. It clogs up the colon, and that directly blocks the performance of the brain. The body is dehydrated and depleted, what leads to chronic anxiety and aggression.

Fat sedates.

Above all, fat consumption makes one want to sit down and not move. It is pacifying and grounding. This of course is very useful to society. Imagine, if we all were constantly moving, running, jumping, having sex, dancing, walking, swimming, climbing trees,...etc. We would be just too wild. No kid would be able to sit through the class. Nobody would stand still in the church, and no one would volunteer for a corporate job.

Imagine, apes at the zoo. What would happen to them if the zoo keepers would all of a sudden decide to feed them eggs, bacon, milk, and peanut butter. "Monkeys!! No more fruit from today on! Sorry! From today on, you eat steak, sausages, cheese, butter, eggs, mayo. Cakes, deserts, whipped cream, ice-cream, chicken soup. Nuts, seeds, oils, avocados. Here you go! Have as much as you want!"

What would happen to our jolly playful chimps, orangutans, gibbons, or powerful gorillas, if they were not allowed to eat fruit? Day by day, we would witness our experimental apes sink into depression, and get aggressive. They would develop tumors, diseases and all sorts of disorders.

Is that surprising? Not at all. It's logical.

We human beings are so clever, and come up with so much research and make-believe science to justify our addiction to fat and addiction to disease and suffering. Prof. Ehret coined it:

"The learned have gone so far as to prove that man belongs biologically in the class of meat-eating animals while the descendant theory proves that he belongs to the ape family, who are exclusively fruit-eaters. You can see how ridiculous - contradictory - so called 'science' is.

They reasoned as follows: Muscles, tissues, the entire body's essential substance is protein: therefore this substance must be introduced into the blood in order to build, to grow. In other words, you must eat muscles to build muscles, you must eat protein to build protein, you must eat fat, to build fat, and in the case of a nursing mother, she must drink milk to make milk!

The cow builds flesh, tissues, bones, hair, milk, efficiency, heat, all from grass exclusively. Feeding milk to a cow to increase milk production would be classed as the height of folly, and yet man does this very thing with himself.

Animal foods cannot build good blood; in fact, do not build human blood at all, because of the biological fact that man is by nature a fruit eater. Look at the juice of a ripe blackberry, black cherry or black grape. Doesn't it almost resemble your blood? Can any reasonable man prove that half decayed 'muscle tissues' build better blood".

We are fooled to believe sugar is bad, and frightened by the warnings that sugar is what causes disease. It is a lie. Sugar is not what's killing us. Fruit sugar especially. It is nothing but bliss, and the closest to mother's milk. Fruit when boiled and melted dissolves into a sirup, molasses, and it is loaded with minerals. You can dilute it in water and fast on it for days! It will give you energy. Raw turbinado cane sugar is just dehydrated cane sugar juice. It is not what's causing disease of the body. Beet sugar, when refined by food industry, becomes white sugar. Yes. It is not the best to eat, but – if you do – it goes right through you. In and out. Firing some hyper vibes in the brain, which seize quickly.

Try eating animal flesh, milk, cheese, oil, butter, avocado and tell me how long is it going to stay in your body. You don't know. That's the problem. The body tissues are like sponge. The fat tends to clog it up, and cause perpetual inflammation and constipation.

Try living on fat. Try making fat the one and only substance you eat. Anthony B. Serna challenges athletes who believe in fat. "Eat a big bowl of avocados and try to run a Marathon!." Anthony runs 14 miles daily and attributes his stamina to intermittent fasting and fruit only nutrition. "I prefer to have a bowl of oranges just before I run! " He used to be 210lbs, depressed, anxious, aggressive, and alcoholic. Today, he says cleansing, fruit, and zero fat is the secret ingredient behind his joyful abstinence and athletic performance. "Fruit is what we humans really crave. It is the secret desire behind all substance addiction – be it alcohol, or drugs. We desire high. We seek energy. We look for the joy and euphoria that fruit supplies in abundance!" According to him, one can overcome any addiction by cleansing, detoxing and overeating fruit.

Anthony says: "The food industry is using sugar to make you eat fat. Otherwise, let's face it, who would buy chocolate? Chocolate is mostly a cacao paste thick as candle wax. Would you eat that? Do you salivate when you look at it? Well... When they add sugar to it, or some sweetener, you will delight in chocolate and get hooked on fat. Just because it has been sweetened to fool you. Raw or not raw is a detail here. Fat content remains the same. It blocks the liver. Sugar is what sells it, what pushes it down the throat. Let's face it, who the heck would eat a birthday cake if it was not sweet!? Why would you? There is nothing fun in eating butter!"

The parasites in the human body have so totally possessed the intelligence of the host and seized control over its brain and nervous impulses, fantasies and cravings, that human beings crave fat - the food supply for parasites, and no longer desire food that nourishes them, the fruit of the orchard. and no longer can digest it easily either. The body clogged up by fat consumption since childhood is getting irritated when fruit comes into the digestive track. It often causes tingling and heart burn, and irritation because fruit acts like a brush inside the body. It sweeps everything on its way. Fruit gets blamed for the discomfort, but not the hot-dog that was eaten the day before. This is why cleansing, detoxing, and juice feasting is so essential to help them body unclog and open it up again to absorb what's good and healthy. As you cleanse, you realize, the more you eat human food - read: fruit - the better you feel. Once you quit eating food of other species, you heal.

Cows milk is for baby cow. It is not yours. Nuts are for squirrels. Grains are for birds. Honey belongs to the bees. Eggs belong to the hens. Animal flesh is not for us to eat. We are not predators or vultures.

Arnold Ehret explains:

"Meat decomposes into pus. Just as soon as the animal is killed the flesh is more or less in decomposition. They are put thru the destructive process of cooking. No meat-eating animal can remain healthy on cooked meat; they must eat it fresh and raw blood, bones and all."

Consider.... If pig's organs are used for medical transplants, because the human body can recognize them and assimilate them as if they were its own, should humans really eat ham? Should humans eat animals if animal flesh looks just like human? Does it not border-line with cannibalism? What will people do if there is no meat in the stores?

Parasites fool you to crave fat. They live in an environment that is filled with mucus, pus and fermentation. They live in anaerobic world - where there is no oxygen, because they produce their own oxygen. This is how cancer sets in.

Parasites get annoyed when you eat fruit, because fruit brings hydration, oxygenation and fiber that brushes them out. Their 'home' becomes uncomfortable. They have to leave your body or die. Don't be surprised if you ever pass worms. Expect it!

Food industry is evolving and morphing. From mainstream supermarket diet, we are moving into more sophisticated vegetarian dishes, vegan menus, and raw gourmet recipes. This is where it gets tricky.

The vegan food movement is very excited to sell you on cruelty-free alternatives, recommending soy products, when you decided to quit eating animals. Bravo for the effort. However, soy is completely indigestible. The body just doesn't know what to do with it, and it's very hard to pass through and discharge. You might as well eat tires with some spices on them! Replacing cow cheese with almond cheese is cruelty-free, but will not lead you to the health level you deserve. Have you ever seen almond cheese growing on trees?

All of vegetarian, vegan and raw vegan menus contain fat. All of them are a lie to the human body, and human nutrition. It's about selling you more products, more stuff and driving you away from the fearless simplicity of life that comes from eating fruit and gentle leafy greens.

Raw food movement is getting increasing popularity. Raw gurus have become successful businessmen. Raw chefs vie on social media showing of their recipes, seasoned with magic powders, and magic potions. All those recipes are based on highfat content. There is maybe a handful of culinary artists today who deliberately create fat free menus, and let's be honest it's hard to show of when all ingredients you have are fresh fruit and veggies.

It's hard to become a multi-millionaire selling fresh fruit and veggies online. Fresh organic produce is one of the worst businesses to be in. Fruit and veggies just get spoiled to quickly! It's so much easier to sell products that will stay fresh for a long time in industrial fridges, or can be dehydrated. Dehydrate goji berries and you can ship them from Himalayas, and tell people they are a healing miracle.

Why Fruit is So Good

Fruit makes your mouth water. That's already a sign your body naturally craves it. It is sensual pleasure for your tongue and the healthiest food you can eat, Chimp!

Coming off the fast is the key to a successful cleanse. If you fasted for seven days, your digestive system is sleeping. If you want to drive the "car", you need to wake up the engine slowly. The way to do it is with fruit, which is juicy, healthy and yummy!

Mouth Watering

Are you salivating? You should be. Have you noticed your mouth is watering when you look at beautiful fruit?

Does your mouth salivate when you look at a cow, or a pig? Are you salivating seeing a fish swimming in the river? Or corn husks? Or a sheaf of rice? Or kale and cabbage? Probably not.

But it does salivate when you look at juicy fruit, which is why fruit is the first and foremost staple of human diet. Fruit is the superfood.

Here's why I eat fruit.

My Body Likes It

I wasn't born vegan, or a raw foodist, or this or that. I have no point of view about food. No ideology or religion. I listen to my body. Ultimately, my body is my only authority. After all, it is the temple of my spirit.

I am spoiled. I like to eat well, and I like to give my body what it requires and desires.

I noticed my body likes fruit. Especially, yummy, juicy tropical fruit. In all the colors, shapes, and flavors. Watermelons cleanse the kidneys, and improve eyesight. Mangos are naturally laxative. Forest berries are simply bliss. As well as savory tomatoes, cucumbers, red peppers, celery, zucchini, etc. I love all varieties, and I shop like a fruit maniac.

You should see me at a Farmers' Market! I buy in bulk!

• Easy To Grow & Harvest

I wasn't born with the eyes that have peripheral vision like the hunting animals do, or ears that can hear from afar, or hunter's claws and fangs. I wasn't born to kill. Not that there is anything wrong with that. Life is a cycle of death and rebirth. It's just not in my nature to have to kill something in order to eat it. And, since I wouldn't kill it, I do not economically participate in the occult practices of the society that sacrifices billions of animals, exposes them into despicable torture, and denies what's going on.

I wasn't born with an oven to bake the foods, or a stove to cook it, or a fridge to store it. I wasn't even born with a dehydrator or a juicer, if we are to apply the same standard of simplicity.

However, I was born with everything I need with which to harvest my food. When I walk into an orchard or a garden, my hands can pick fruit easily and naturally, put it into my mouth, and - most of the time - I don't even need a knife to open it. My teeth can go right inside. My food grows abundantly everywhere, and does not require much labor to harvest it.

• Instantly Digested & Assimilated

Digestion of fruit is effortless, and instantaneous. Have you noticed? Wake up, and instead of coffee in the morning, have a slice of watermelon. Within a couple of seconds you will feel energy shooting into your brain. This occurs if your blood vessels and tissues are not clogged up by fat. They shouldn't be after the fasting you did, and they won't unless you start eating oils, nuts and seeds. (Not to mention animal products!)

Fruit is juicy! The more juicy it is, the better for you. And the quality of the water inside a fruit is the best in the world. The tree in order to produce fruit had to pull the water through its roots, trunk, branches and twigs. The best carbon filter ever! The water in fruit has tiny molecules which easily penetrate the brain barrier, while - for example - water in plastic bottles doesn't.

Dehydrated fruit never carries the same benefits as fresh one. Anything that's dehydrated is no longer 'whole food, and it is constipating. You will need to hydrated it, soak it, in order to absorb it, or it will drain water out of your own body and dehydrate you in the process.

My friend and colonic hydrotherapist, Desiree Huizar Wilson, says: "If you can't squeeze it in your hand, it's going to make you constipated." Do you know why? Because intestines work very hard squeezing out all the juices and pushing out the rest! It is called peristaltic movement.

Alkaline, Antioxidant, Structured

Water contained in fresh organic fruit carrying alkaline minerals, antioxidants, and it is naturally structured in crystals. That water is evaporated when you dehydrate foods. Gone, together with a whole bunch of health benefits, and the capacity to super-hydrate your brain. When I eat fruit, my mind is sharp, and I have lots of energy!

If you cut fruit in half you will see structure inside. You will see symmetry and beauty. You will also see the glitter of sunlight in it. It often makes me think of the beautiful water crystals of Masaru Emoto. For billions of years the same drops of water have been circulating on the Earth. Every drop of water carries the memory of our ancient history on the Planet, and its trees. Thus fruit is the hope for our liberation.

Brain-Food, and Brain-Hydration

Fruit is the magic superfood that powers the brain. Mainstream dietitians will tell you to avoid fruit, and guess what happens when you do? You end up eating sugar. That is because your brain needs simple carbohydrates to function like the supercomputer that it is.

Simple carbs can come from whole, organic fruits, and they will be instantly absorbed into the bloodstream and rapidly carried into the brain, provided there is nothing blocking that process.

And when in a fat-coated digestive tract, fruit doesn't get digested; rather, it ferments in the intestine, feeding candida, which when overgrown, destabilizes the brain chemistry, causing emotional imbalance.

Your brain needs water to process all the complicated neurotransmissions that go on inside.

Most bottled water on the market is acidic, due to the petroleum-based chemicals leaking from plastic. If you test it with pH drops, you will see it will turn out orange, or yellow at best.

Spring water from Fiji may be a nice idea in Fiji, but before it gets over to you, it's spring water plus petroleum, which makes it very acidic. ORP (Oxidation Reduction Potential) meters show it is also highly oxidizing; that means it will contribute to more free radicals in your blood and make you age faster.

No matter how much you drink of this water, your brain will be dehydrated like a dried nut. That may show up as depression, fogginess, lack of concentration, weight imbalance, and moodiness, and some believe we see it in children as autism, ADD, ADHD, OCD, etc.

• **Weight Loss & Sports Performance**

If you are thinking weight loss, think fruit. If you are thinking muscles, think fruit. Fruit is the magic behind the victories of the Olympians.

If you are interested to champion your life, go fruit yourself! It is the simplest jungle diet you can imagine. Add some tender leafy greens, make salads or eat mono-meals, and have fun!

There are two principle sources of energy on the Planet that are embodied in fruit – the energy of the sun and the energy of water. It is also bathed in wind which is the third source of power on the Earth. What if your body is a sports vehicle? Would you like to power it up?

It is an irony to hear doctors and nutritionists telling people not to eat fruit. Sure! Avoid fruit and you will end up bingeing on stuff loaded with white sugar and corn syrup. It is a joke to hear wellness experts and raw food gurus lecture on the dangers of fruit, when they should be the first ones teaching people to plant fruit trees. Instead, they recommend menus that are mostly nuts, avocados and cacao. If you study the ingredients, you will understand why every meal in a raw food restaurant swimming in fat. Virtually every smoothie, soup, main course, salad dressing, and desert. People dine there believing they are eating healthy, and yet when they return home they feel constipated and bloated. The ideal of raw food being superior is destroyed by the density of what they consumed. So what that it hasn't been exposed to temperature? If you partake on daily basis in this lifestyle, do not be surprised to develop acid reflux, yeast infections, etc; to begin with... If you purify your body by cleansing and eating fruit for a while, your instincts will awaken. Your body will instantly reject any kind of fat or poison like cacao. It will simply vomit everything out.

Swami Sri Yukteswar, the spiritual master of Yogananada, in his book 'The Holy Science', teaches how to distinguish which foods are natural to human species:

In men of all races we find that their senses of smell, sound, and sight never lead them to slaughter animals; on the contrary they cannot bear even the sight of such killings. Slaughter houses are always recommended to be removed far from the towns: men often pass strict ordinances forbidding the uncovered transportation of flesh meats. Can flesh then be considered the natural food of man, when both his eyes and his nose are so much against it, unless deceived by flavors of spices, salt, and sugar? On the other hand, how delightful do we find the fragrance of fruits, the very sight of which often makes the mouth water! It may also be noticed that various grains and roots posses an agreeable odor and taste, though faint, even when unprepared. Thus again, we are led to infer from these observations that man was intended to be a frugivorous animals.

Other foods are unnatural to man and being uncongenial to the system are necessarily foreign to it; when they enter the stomach, they are not properly assimilated. Missed with the blood, they accumulate in the excretory and other organs not properly adapted to them. When they cannot find their way out, they subside in tissue crevices by the law of gravitation; and, being fermented, produce, diseases, mental and physical, and ultimately lead to premature death.

Experiment also proves that the nonirritant diet natural to the vegetarian is, almost without exception, admirably suited to children's development, both physical and mental. Their minds, understanding, will, the principal faculties, temper, and general disposition are also properly developed.

In the Genesis, it is said Adam and Eve ate fruit and herbs. However, today, majority of human beings are eating fat from tortured animals. It shows how far we have gone astray, while Eden is still here on the Earth. It is just poisoned, and polluted. It is up to us to reclaim it. Fruit is the way back to Eden. It is what makes life juicy and fertile. It shifts our consciousness back to that of freedom and abundance.

We human beings are symbiotic with Trees. We breath in oxygen they make, and breath out carbon dioxide they need. Trees provide us with shade to enjoy, and wood for making shelter and furniture. When we eat fruit, we heal. It's impossible to overdose it. Worst comes to worse - you poop - which in Nature would help to grow more trees!

Ever since Eve ate the apple, fruit has been forbidden on the Planet. We have created a civilization against pleasure, especially against the pleasure of women, and a culture of fancy culinary recipes, all of which unsuccessfully attempt to replace the sweet delight of fruit, and succeed at bringing suffering, while man is hoping to reach heaven after painful death.

Why I Am Nuts for Coconuts

Since I lived in the Hawaiian Islands, I found a way to cleanse with raw organic coconut water. The secret grows on the tree!

Open a coconut, and drink as much you feel like! Try it next time you are on a tropical voyage!

Your belly will get full pretty fast, so no worries, you can't possibly overdose on coconuts. Coconuts vary in size and flavor of water, so it might be a different number for you, if you are, for example, drinking Thai organic cocos. In any case - drink! Stay hydrated!

Here are some of the benefits or fresh raw organic coconut water. Once you taste the flavor, you will never settle for any looka-like product from a carton box or a can. It doesn't even compare!

Coconut water is alkaline

Its biochemical composition is the closest to human blood.

In fact, it is the only natural liquid you can inject into veins. Therefore, cleansing on coconut water is like having a "liquid blood transfusion". During World War II when blood supplies were running low, doctors discovered that the liquid inside young coconuts could be used as a substitute for blood plasma. India's National Newspaper, November 24, 2003 states:

"It (coconut juice) is also considered a close substitute for blood plasma since it is sterile, cool, easily absorbed by the body and does not destroy red blood cells. To quote Morton Satin, Chief of Food and Agricultural Organization's Agricultural Industries and Post Harvest Management Service: 'It is a natural isotonic beverage with the same level of electrolytic balance as we have in our blood. It is the fluid of life, so to speak."

Coconut water is nutritious

It is very low in fat. You can drink as much as you want without worrying about over-indulging. It's full of nutrients and minerals that help you feel full, thus decreasing your cravings for excessive foods. You are being nourished on a cellular level, so you don't feel hungry during the cleanse. It is also yummy!

Coconut water is super-hydrating

It has more hydrating properties than bottled spring water, so drinking it can certainly help your digestion. Thus, you'll be able to absorb food nutrients better and have easier bowel movements. It is also structured in small molecules, which allows it to enter your body cells and provide hydration.

Coconut water boosts the immune system

Coconut water has anti-viral and anti-fungal properties that can help you avoid disease in the body and boost your immune system. It creates an alkaline environment, which becomes unbearable to the microbes that proliferate when the body liquids are acidic. Medical research on the healing benefits of coconut water is astounding.

Coconut water is revitalizing

It contains less sodium and more potassium than the average energy or sports drink. It is a highly desirable substitute for these expensive and artificial products, which might explain the booming coconut drink industry, even though the coconut water sold in cans and boxes is pasteurized (not raw).

Coconut water is full of electrolytes

Electrolytes are biochemicals that help to absorb minerals. Coconut has so many of these ions that it is often recommended for hangover relief or as a sports drink. It is also great for headaches and mood balancing.

Coconut water is magical

This is my subjective experience. I've noticed there is something magical about a coconut. It opens psychic abilities and facilitates manifestation more than any other liquid. Perhaps it is why the native people consider wherever coconuts grow to be sacred.

Nature comes with its natural container. The coconut water when it's raw is packaged in nothing else but the shell. Organic coconuts are the ones that have not been washed in formaldehyde. Ask your provider!

Modern medical science is now confirming the use of coconut in treating many conditions. Published studies in medical journals show that coconut in one form or another may provide a wide range of health benefits. Some of these are summarized below by the Coconut Research Center, established in Colorado by Dr. Bruce Fife, N.D., the author of Coconut Cures: Preventing and Treating Common Health Problems with Coconut:

- Kills viruses that cause influenza, herpes, measles, hepatitis C, SARS, AIDS, and other illnesses.

- Kills bacteria that cause ulcers, throat infections, urinary tract infections, gum disease and cavities, pneumonia, and gonorrhea, and other diseases.

- Kills fungi and yeasts that cause candidiasis, ringworm, athlete's foot, thrush, diaper rash, and other infections.

- Expels or kills tapeworms, lice, giardia and other parasites.

- Provides a nutritional source of quick energy.

- Boosts energy and endurance, enhancing physical and athletic performance.

- Improves digestion and absorption of other nutrients including vitamins, minerals, and amino acids.

- Improves insulin secretion and utilization of blood glucose.

- Relieves stress on pancreas and enzyme systems of the body.

- Reduces symptoms associated with pancreatitis.

- Helps relieve symptoms and reduce health risks associated with diabetes.

- Reduces problems associated with malabsorption syndrome and cystic fibrosis.

- Improves calcium and magnesium absorption and supports the development of strong bones and teeth.

- Helps protect against osteoporosis.

- Helps relieve symptoms associated with gallbladder disease.

- Relieves symptoms of Crohn's disease, ulcerative colitis, and stomach ulcers.

- Improves digestion and bowel function.

- Relieves pain and irritation caused by hemorrhoids.

- Reduces inflammation.

- Supports tissue healing and repair.

- Supports and aids immune system function.

- Helps protect the body from breast, colon, and other cancers.

- Is heart healthy; improves cholesterol ratio, reducing risk of heart disease.
- Protects arteries from injury that causes atherosclerosis and thus protects against heart disease.
- Helps prevent periodontal disease and tooth decay.
- Functions as a protective antioxidant.
- Helps to protect the body from harmful free radicals that promote premature aging and degenerative disease.
- Does not deplete the body's antioxidant reserves like other oils do.
- Improves utilization of essential fatty acids and protects them from oxidation.
- Helps relieve symptoms associated with chronic fatigue syndrome.
- Relieves symptoms associated with prostate enlargement.
- Reduces epileptic seizures.
- Dissolves kidney stones.
- Helps prevent liver disease.
- Is lower in calories than all other fats.
- Supports thyroid function.
- Promotes loss of excess weight by increasing metabolic rate.
- Is utilized by the body to produce energy vs. being stored as body fat like other dietary fats.
- Helps prevent obesity.
- Applied topically, helps to form a chemical barrier on the skin to ward off infection.
- Reduces symptoms associated with psoriasis, eczema, and dermatitis.
- Supports the natural chemical balance of the skin.
- Prevents wrinkles, sagging skin, and age spots.
- Promotes healthy looking hair and complexion.
- Helps control dandruff.

- Provides protection from damaging effects of ultraviolet radiation from the sun.
- Does not form harmful by-products when heated to normal cooking temperature like other vegetable oils do.
- Has no harmful or discomforting side effects.
- Is completely nontoxic to humans.

No Cocos? Go Juicing!

Coconut water fasting is one of the most difficult cleanses you will do. So, before you jump into it, you might want to do a couple of juice fasts at home to prepare your body. Juice Granny Smith apples throughout the first three days of your cleanse, adding some ginger. If you drink two tall glasses, every two hours, it's going to move things in your body - oooooh! - like nothing else. Apple juice has a high concentration of mallic acid, which opens your body tissues, and helps to soften the gallbladder stones and release them. It can give you diarrhea or make you nauseous. Granny Smith apple juice fast was the original Max Gerson Therapy . This is how Dr Max Gerson healed himself and other people around him. It's a powerful liver flush!

If you find the apple juice treatment too hard on your body, you can add some carrots to make it more soothing for you. You can drink some orange juice from time to time, or interchange Red Juice and Green Juice throughout the day.

Red Juice is beets, carrots, Fuji apples, lime or lemon, and ginger.

Green Juice is cucumber, kale, celery, Granny Smith apples, lime, and ginger.

It will be great for purifying your blood, and more gentle on the body. You can make many different combinations when juicing fruits and veggies.

Get creative. Play. Drink, drink, and drink! Any time you are hungry, drink.

Any time you are thirsty, wait! Don't even let your body get there! If you are thirsty, you are already dehydrated. So, drink before you become thirsty! Stay hydrated.

Did I say already: if you don't have a juicer, sell your car?! If you have a juicer, what are you waiting for?

***

Yes! Totally Anti-Social!

Note: Eating for your body may be considered politically incorrect. After all, the majority of society is eating to create disease, high medical bills and something to talk about at family reunions. If you choose a lifestyle that is marked by health, happiness and consciousness, you might lose friends.

They will host a dinner at their home; you will bring your own food. They will invite you to a restaurant; you will be fussy and picky. They will serve coffee and you won't drink it. They will want to please you with raw chocolate and you might feel compelled to give them a lecture on what it does to the liver. They will eat ice cream around you, and you won't even salivate.

You will see people dying slowly, digging their grave with their teeth, and they will be upset with you for refusing to join them. You will be told their food is cheap, and you spend too much.

Well, who owns you? Who owns your body? What if you unplug and become free? How wild, healthy and dangerous are you going to be?

What if you being you is going to be so contagious that people around you are going to start choosing more for them? What if you being you is going to cause discomfort? And what if the biggest changes are possible when there is discomfort?

What if your choices bring on judgment? And, what if every time they judge you they give you energy? What if judgment brings money? What if you being vibrantly healthy and joyous is going to be so contagious that people will throw money at you?

How To Live a Healthy Life

Living a healthy life is way easier and cheaper than living a life of misery, obesity and disease. In the former you profit. In the latter something alien profits from you.

Go ahead. Reclaim your body!

It's unbelievable how much stuff we carry inside our bodies and live with, walk around with, participate in sports with, go shopping with, have sex with, watch TV with, etc. It's unthinkable how our bodies rot inside, while we spend tons of money fixing cars, chasing fashion, wearing make-up, and so on. It's admirable how our bodies can accumulate toxins in certain organs, and keep them sequestered "off the beaten path" so that we can function, no matter what.

Have you noticed some people have a better relationship with their pets than with their bodies? American people have a better relationship with their cars than with their bodies. They know how to change oil in the car, or fix a tire, or flush their carburetor, but they have no clue about how to cleanse their colon or do a liver flush. The same people would get furious if their mechanic took out a part of their car without replacing it, while they are okay with their doctor cutting out their gallbladder, or replacing their stomach with a plastic bag.

Cleansing is all about resetting your relationship with your body. It's all about you reclaiming your body and, as a result, every area of your life. Fasting is just a vehicle for this to take place. So is eating healthily.

Ultimately, if you judge yourself, and if you judge your body, if you continue the guilt-blame-shame game that perpetuates disease on this planet - nothing will really shift. No cleansing, fasting, juicing, or the most sophisticated diet will make an impact. It's all in you being you and choosing more for you, and honoring your body with the most yummy, nutritious meals it desires and requires. It's your body that's eating - not you.

What if you asked your body: "What would you like to have?"

I am not an expert on your body. I am an expert on my own body though, and I am sharing with you what has worked with me. If you apply it in your life, you might discover you can be an expert on your own body, too.

Unless you have kids, you are responsible for one life only - your own. If you have given control over your own life to someone else, you will need to reclaim it in order to heal yourself. Be it your mother-in-law, TV commercials, your spouse or your boss. It is only after you reclaim your own life that you will be able to give it away - to a cause that truly inspires you, and carries you in the world, and it will become your greatest source of joy.

There is a way for you to be in this world and be not of this world. This world is so toxic and so sticky that you will need to use fasting as a way of regular purification, regrouping, and regaining your sense of who you are and where you are going.

Like me, you may discover that cleansing is a lifestyle. It is like brushing your teeth, taking a shower, or taking a vacation from work. You might love it so much that you will do it several times a year - Spring and Autumn - renewing yourself like Nature, or whenever you feel you need to say good-bye to a relationship and cleanse, shed-ding a skin like a snake.

Today, I can tell you cleansing might be a lot easier for your body than keeping all the toxic crap inside, carrying it around the world, and feeling sick and tired.

Feeling light is just way more fun! What's terrifying to you is the idea of moving towards the unknown, letting go, and the rite of passage you will need to go through to transform.

Here is a little summary of what I hope you have learned in this book, and seven tips for successfully moving into a healthy way of living:

• Say Good-bye to the Old You

What if you, your body, and your life are never going to be the same? Who says you are the same today as you were yesterday, anyways? Isn't your body constantly changing? The trillion gazillion cells? The Universe is constantly changing, and you are embarking on a journey that's going to shift your reality. So how about saying good-bye to everything that's no longer working for you?

Make a list: "What am I saying good-bye to?"

Take full responsibility for what you have created. If you have created it, you are the one who can destroy and uncreate it. You are the one who can create something new. That's how creative you are!

We are accustomed to resist change. We bought into an idea that change must be horrible, mean and awful. What if change is fun? What if change is easy? What if change is natural, and organic?

• Rise Before the Sun

Something magical happens when you rise early. You and your body catch the energy of the Sun, which is the source of energy on the planet.

As you do it daily, as you introduce it into your lifestyle, you will tap into the morphogenetic field of the Earth.

I notice that when I rise before sunrise, it rejuvenates me, creates abundant miracles in my day, and all of a sudden, I've got all kinds of time! I find I can easily accomplish everything I need to do during the day. I also find time to write down my dreams, which helps me to remember them, and access a different plane of reality.

What if you moved all the work you normally do in the evening to the morning?

Did you know that many of the outstanding people in history, all the greatest leaders of consciousness, would wake up before sunrise?

What is it going to contribute to you?

What if you discover your mind is crystal clear, and you are able to get everything done with ease, joy, and glory, when you rise early?

• Go to Sleep Early

Have you noticed that electricity has been invented only recently?

For thousands of years, we were going to sleep at dusk, and only recently have we shifted our schedule into a nightlife of surfing the Internet, partying, doing business, watching TV, etc.

Is there any research on how our bodies are affected by this?

The adrenal cortex hormone and growth hormone are secreted during the night during sleep. The former, which can promote the metabolism of carbohydrates in the body, and protect the development of muscle, is secreted before dawn, while the latter is produced only after sleep, and can delay the aging process.

The period between 11 p.m. and 3 a.m. the next day is the beauty time, and it is also the time for the meridians in the human body to move and activate the gallbladder and liver. If these two organs do not have adequate rest, it will be reflected on the skin.

Problems such as roughness, yellowish face, dark spots and acne will appear. What's worse, the long-term practice of staying up late will slowly cause some neurological and psychiatric symptoms such as insomnia, forgetfulness, irritability, anxiety and so on.

The Chinese, who have studied the human body for centuries, found that each organ has a particular clock. They say that your liver, which is the largest organ of your body, starts working at 9 p.m. in the summer, and at 8 p.m. in the winter. It goes to work when you rest.

The liver rotates your blood within your body, and purifies it. Sleeping early will support your liver in alkalizing and rebuilding your blood. When your blood is pure, you and your entire body feel rested, energized and rejuvenated. Do it, and see for yourself!

If you have trouble going to sleep early, no problem! Set an alarm clock at 5 a.m. for a few days in a row, and I guarantee you will be sleeping like a baby soon after sunset.

You will benefit from this habit, especially if you wish to rejuvenate. It's absolutely essential to get to bed early when you are healing from a disease.

• Alkalize your Blood

It takes only three days for your blood to turn from acid into alkaline. Only three days! Most people give up on Day 2, because they feel awful. They have no idea that if they go through the first three days, Day 4 already feels better, Day 5 feels amazing, and Day 6, you might have energy through the roof!

The detox side effects can be similar to the symptoms of flu. You may have headaches, dizziness, fever, shivers, diarrhea, etc.

The blood pH is turning from acid to alkaline, and to your body this is a bit like an express train heading to NYC and all of a sudden switching gears to go back to LA. It just throws your body up in the air, releasing a lot of toxic residue into the bloodstream.

Once you get through the first three days, you will be surprised how much easier it gets afterwards.

On the other hand, what if your body is detoxifying when you have the flu?

There is no difference. During the cleanse you are just choosing to do it consciously!

The simplest way to alkalize your blood is to choose happiness. That doesn't come easy if your body is toxic. Your brain might be just stuck somewhere else, processing the biochemical addiction to suffering, and playing it over and over like a broken record. How much fun is there in that?

Another simple technique is to over-eat fruit. Try it! It's impossible! And the result is... Euphoria!

• Forgive Radically

I have not yet met anyone healthy who has not forgiven. And you? Have you seen anyone who holds grudges, and is truly radiantly, vigorously, contagiously healthy? This does not happen.

If you would truly like to cleanse and push the reset buttons on everything in your life, - your body, mind, spirit, past, present, future, and all the seven chakras, the infinite being you are - you need to forgive.

The question is: How will you know you have forgiven? I often hear: "I forgave. It's the past. I let go." Somehow, I do not sense an abundance of joy in that.

What if everything that happened to you happened for you? How grateful would you be? What if there is nothing to forgive? What if it is only your judgment of the situation? Nothing short of gratitude is a sign of true forgiveness.

• Question Everything

What if everything you have ever been told about you and your body is a lie?

What if all the ways you were told you should be, all the stuff you heard from your parents, school, television, all the stuff "They" say, is just an interesting point of view?

Dr. Dain Heer in his book, Being You, Changing the World, poses these questions: "What if you being you is what the world requires to change? What would it take for you to realize how crucial you are to possibilities of the world?"

Cleansing will require you to critically examine your life. From where you function, all your relationships, what's really working for you, and what's not. A bit like a plumber who enters the kitchen when it's flooded. You will need to check every "pipe" to see where your energy is leaking, and seal it right there. This will require you to examine every answer you have been told in your life.

If answers were the solution to your problems, shouldn't you have solved them a long time ago? Did you not get enough answers by now?

What if you ask: "What else is possible? What's great about me that I am just not seeing? How does it get any better than this?"

What if you live in wonder? What if you be the question, as opposed to trying to be the answer and trying to get it always right?

• Choose Joy!

What if you are here to have fun? What if things are not right or wrong, good or bad? What if there is only choice, and what would it take for you to choose what brings you joy?

Do you know what gives you joy? Maybe it is a type of movement that your body requires: yoga, dance, walking? Maybe it is a kind of fragrance: a flower, essential oils? A certain fengshui space arrangement in your home? What kind of colors? What kind of touch? What else would you add into your life?

Oops! You weren't supposed to know that you are here to have fun! That changes the whole system, doesn't it?

Natural Hygiene

Of all the crazy-weird stuff I do, simple natural hygiene is probably one of the most surprising. Other than for photo shoots, or if I am on TV or filming a movie, or at a party, I do not use cosmetics. Yeah, zero. They are acidic. Did you know? So they would age my skin.

Instead, I scrub my body with sea-salt, use hot-cold-hotcold showers interchangeably, and sometimes I like to put organic clay on my face as a mask. Nothing like encountering Mother Earth - face-to-face!

Instead of using toothpaste, I make my own with baking soda or clay, or simply rub my teeth and gums with the white side of an orange peel or banana peel. I paid a visit a special dentist to remove my amalgam feelings which contained mercury.

I do not use soaps, shampoo, or hair products that foam. I do not use a deodorant at all, since I do not stink. I use special filters on the shower and tap to remove fluoride. Few dare to question its usage, besides the obvious purpose of pacification of the mind. I do not feel like being pacified.

How to Reach for Greatness

The quality of your life depends not on the answers you have, but on the questions you ask.

Keep asking: What else is possible? Keep pushing the envelope.

Have you noticed that I ask a lot of questions? I have no answers for you. All I have are questions that are going to expand your infinite possibilities, and give you more choice. Isn't that what questions do? In either case, do not believe me, or anything you hear in this world. What if 98% of this reality is based on an illusion? Check for yourself. Find your own answers within your own body.

Instead of seeking answers in your life, ask more questions during your cleanse. Questions are like windows for your mind to expand, be free and explore. Through them you can see a world of possibilities. You can open them, and let the fresh air come in.

Many life coaches today realize that answers disempower us, while questions can truly empower us to seek and find on our own. Coaching in the form of questions is known in Buddhism as "koan". The Buddhist masters would pose questions to their students as opposed to giving them answers.

According to Asian medical systems, there are seven energy vortexes in the body and they are called the chakras. They run all along the spinal column from the bottom to the top of the head. Even though Western medicine has not proved their existence, it has not disproved it either - especially since the seven chakras seem to correspond with our seven hormonal glands. They bring energy to different body organs and they also reflect our belief system.

The seven chakras are root chakra, sex or sacral chakra, solar plexus, heart chakra, throat chakra, third eye chakra, and the crown chakra. Just like someone's heart can be closed, or someone's mind can be lacking vision, in the same way all the other "energy centers" of the body react to our thoughts, feelings and emotions. Thus, our body is constantly bathing in the "aura" of our thoughts, feelings and emotions, which ultimately constitute our immune system.

We all have free will. Nothing can take it away from us, but our free will functions based on our beliefs - the stuff we've taken for granted as answers. We got them from parents, religion, society, school, media, etc. Have you noticed? We have inherited lots of limiting points of view that no longer serve us. We bought into a lot of garbage and lies about our body, healing, money, and sexuality. Successful leaders in the world have rejected most of these beliefs long ago. For some reason these limiting beliefs continue to be spoon-fed to the masses, even though they are utterly unscientific. See what happens when you apply questions each day, chakra by chakra.

Here's a way for you to question all that programing, and do a seven-day detox of your mind. You can do it while you are fasting and juicing. It will be super powerful! This way you get to change your life, transform it and design it consciously, rather than having it designed and framed for you. Yes. You can choose what you believe. You can choose what point of view works for you!

Do you remember what I said to my doctors? I told them toxic food and toxic thoughts created my illness. Just as food can be acidic, so can your thoughts, burning through your peace, causing mental pain and discomfort. Instead of thinking them through and sifting them out-positive vs. negative, I dump thoughts out of my head altogether. I just simply set my mind on questions. I find questions to be very alkaline, calming and soothing.

Some people believe that happiness is reached through smoking pot. Unfortunately, pot will make your blood acidic. It will also leave you dehydrated and hungry. Marijuana is extremely yin, so it will make your body crave foods that are extremely yanf: salt, meat, cheese, eggs, bread, etc. It is also very addictive. If used long term, it will destroy your body and your mind.

Today more and more doctors are recommending marijuana for all sorts of symptoms, starting with depression. Depression is a symptom of a blocked liver and sluggish blood. Marijuana will only mask the symptoms for a short while, and make one temporarily feel good. It is not going to be enough to flush the gallstones and purify the blood. Pot may be fun shortterm. It is receiving huge amounts of press and publicity today as the panacea for all. The substance is used by so many of my vegan friends it is almost unpopular to question it, especially when it has been "recommended by a doctor". Some doctors prescribe painkillers based on opium or synthetic heroin. They prescribe a drug derived from amphetamine to children that don't fit into our crazy world. Does that make these doctors right?

Even though we may see headlines on CNN: "Marijuana stops child's severe seizures", one may ask what caused them? Maybe the child would not have any seizures at all if given plenty of organic fruit at home and in the school instead of meat, wheat, dairy, and corn syrup?!

CBD oil? The body instantly feels better, right? Question: Why is that? Maybe because it has been poisoned and it needs to mobilize all its vitalize forces to neutralize it. Notice, if you cleanse, detox and eat fruit - you wont' need any of that. It's a crutch. An excuse. A pacifier that keeps you from changing things and freeing yourself forever.

According to Dr. Robert O. Young, a microbiologist and biochemist known for his live blood cell analysis, "Using marijuana for medicinal purposes can only lead to increased systemic latent tissue acidosis and the destruction of the alkaline design of the body. Marijuana is acidifying to the blood and tissues and therefore cannot bring balance, harmony, energy or health to the body." If you want to cleanse your body, marijuana is not the path.

Speaking from the standpoint of ancient Indian Yoga and Chinese Martial Arts, nothing should enter your lungs but fresh air. Your lungs, your body and your brain crave oxygen to be on a high. Oxygen carries *prana* (Sanskrit for "life force"), which brings a borderline euphoric state of joy. Marijuana, like any psychedelic, is a way to evade reality.

This reality is completely nuts. Yes. Agreed. However, what if the way out is the way through? Are you ready to claim the power?

Important. Please - this is your homework. Do it for you and just for you. Not for your mother, father, sister, brother, husband, girlfriend. Just for you, so you would know what you choose for yourself in your life.

You may invite them later to play with you - after your cleanse is over - unless they have decided to do the cleanse with you and have joined you in fasting. In that case, you each still do it for you, and then in the evening you can meet and share what this process was like, compare notes, etc. Have a blast!

Day One – Focus on the Root Chakra

This is the day you "root" your cleanse. This is the day to discharge and release what's no longer working for you. Make a list: "To what are you saying 'good-bye'?" Sign it, date it, and burn it before sunset.

Energy healer Cheri Valentine has studied the chakras and writes: "Family wounds and tribal beliefs are stored in the body in this area. Health of this chakra is associated with your upbringing and early life. Changes can be made by examining your family's beliefs and releasing those that limit you. Fear of not being safe is a common block.

"This chakra is your foundation. The basic issues associated with the root chakra are instinct, safety, survival, grounding, family, security, boundaries, and new beginnings."

Day Two – Focus on the Sex Chakra

This is the day you create a new vision. Make a mind-map: "What else is possible? What kind of life would you like to live and create? Can you sense the possibility of a great life for you? What does it feel like?" List all the elements, draw the picture, and make a vision board!

Cheri Valentine: "Beliefs tied to this sacral chakra can be about fear of abandonment, financial security, social status, children, and creativity. You can be controlled by your fears, level of trust, control, blame, guilt and shame. The daily aspects of living, people in our lives, and the quality of our relationships center in this chakra. It also relates to everything we own, money, relationships, and passion.

"Clearing this chakra unblocks our creativity, sexuality, money, relationships, empathy, nurturing, pleasure, emotions, movement, change, warmth, and intimacy. And greatly enhances your ability to go with the flow, living in grace and acceptance and allowing yourself to enjoy your life and achievements."

Day Three – Focus on the Power Chakra

This is the day you identify things in your life that have been blocking your true potential. "To whom does it belong?"

Make a list of all the people who you believe hurt you. Write letters of Radical Forgiveness. Sign, date, and burn.

Cheri Valentine: "This area controls digestion and the metabolic systems that process the energy needed to overcome inertia and apathy, and get us moving from our stuck status.

Also called the Solar Chakra, it is from this center that we assert our personal power, follow our gut instincts, take risks and make decisions. It is where we feel self-respect, confidence, and decisiveness. This is the area of assertiveness, intuition, and inner drive."

Day Four – Focus on the Heart Chakra

This is the day you step into being the Real You. Reflect: "What if you being you is what the world requires to change? What would it take for you to realize what a treasure you are to the possibilities of the world?"

Cheri Valentine: "Many have learned to shut down or close off their hearts to protect themselves, at a tremendous cost of living without love.

The basic issues of your heart chakra are love, compassion, kindness, relationships, self-acceptance, forgiveness, hope, sympathy, and empathy. Opening this center means you are now fully participating in the magic of the Universe."

Day Five – Focus on the Throat Chakra

This is the day you step into what's true for you. Ask: "What brings you joy? What makes you feel inspired? What makes you feel uplifted and empowered?" On this day you learn to relate consciously with your body, and chose to be real instead of being nice.

What if you being real is way more fun?

Cheri Valentine: "Health problems in this area are tied to repressing your feelings, especially anger. It could be that you are holding old emotions from childhood that were never acknowledged.

The throat chakra governs voice, communication, clairaudience, listening, creativity, self-expression, self-image, humility, manifesting ideas, vibration, telepathy, and channeling your own higher wisdom."

Day Six – Focus on the Third Eye

This is the day you learn to trust your own knowing and inner vision. Ask: "What if you know that you know? What if you are your own psychic? What do you know that you are pretending not to know?"

Cheri Valentine: "The basic issues of this chakra are intellect, perception, wisdom, insight, clarity, clairvoyance, imagination, dreams, ideas, reasoning, connection to the higher self and telepathy. This energy center combines the clearly focused left-brain, which computes and analyzes, with an open right-brain, which is where our intuitive, artistic and psychic gifts reside. Opening this chakra teaches you discernment and wisdom, where you can focus on your inner state of awareness and the outer world at the same time. It helps you to see clearly what is important for your own well-being and happiness, giving you a sense of perspective and insight."

Day Seven – Focus on the Crown Chakra

This is the day you design your own reality. Ask: "What if you could be the Master of this reality? What if this reality can work for you? How does it get even better than this?" On this day, you master your magic.

Cheri Valentine: "Your attitude, beliefs, faith, values, conscience, courage and humanitarianism have been developed and represented in this chakra. When you experience lack of purpose, loss of meaning in your life, indifference, and depression, your crown chakra may be unbalanced. Your moral and ethical beliefs may be weak and you may have a high attachment to material needs. You may also feel disconnected from nature and the flow of life. You may either have an unquestioning and rigid following of religious dogma or have no spirituality existent in your life or beliefs.

The basic issues of your crown chakra are connection to Source or the Divine, wisdom, intuitive knowing, spiritual development, selflessness, universal higher consciousness, knowledge, understanding, consciousness, and meditation."

Energy Healing

During your cleanse, you and your body will benefit from various healing modalities that are coming out into the world today. I enjoy various types of massage (especially Hawaiian LomiLomi), sound healing with gongs and Tibetan bowls, the

Plexus Method of Bio-Energy, Rolfing, Matrix Energetics, Craniosacral Massage, etc.

These and many other energy healing modalities are profoundly rejuvenating, detoxifying, and provide resetting buttons on everything we know as reality. They raise the vibration of your personal reality, and thus change the environment your body cells are immersed in. This is one of the most important factors of healing and creating a new lifestyle for you.

The Beast of Cancer

"Cancer does not have a face until it's yours or someone you know".

-Anthony Del Monte

Is cancer a death sentence passed on you, if you buy into it? Is it a marketing brand designed to sell you a treatment plan with chemicals to kill you? Or is it a parasite that breeds on the human body? Or is it an alien demon creeping into one's aura and feeding upon one's fear and sadness, as the shamanic healers would say?

According to Center for Diseases Control, American government agency, "Cancer is the name given to a collection of related diseases". Interesting, isn't it? What does it mean?

In my Polish common sense brain, I knew the cure is the cause. If I stop the cause, I will take the bull by the horns. The definition of insanity, according to Albert Einstein, is to "Keep doing the same things and expect different results". I knew I needed to do something radically different.

My doctors laughed at me when I asked them about the cause of my disease. They said they would get a Nobel Prize if they knew.

Well, there was someone who did!

In 1931, Otto Warburg, a German physiologist and medical doctor, won the Nobel Prize for discovering the cause of cancer.

In his own words:

"Cancer, above all other diseases, has countless secondary causes. But, even for cancer, there is only one prime cause. Summarized in a few words, the prime cause of cancer is the replacement of the respiration of oxygen in normal body cells by a fermentation of sugar."

Wikipedia says:

"The concept that cancer cells switch to fermentation in lieu of aerobic respiration has become widely accepted, even if it is not seen as the cause of cancer. Some suggest the Warburg phenomenon could be used to develop anti-cancer drugs."

So, wait a minute. The cause of cancer has been known for nearly 100 years? And doctors don't know it? The media doesn't talk about it?

In 1958, after thirty years of clinical experimentation, Max Gerson, another German medical doctor, published his book: A Cancer Therapy: Results of 50 Cases. This medical monograph details the theories, treatment, and results achieved by this outstanding, ingenious physician, who practiced what he preached.

Dr. Gerson started by healing himself from debilitating migraines by experimenting with diet. He was surprised to discover that his "migraine diet" also healed his skin tuberculosis. In a carefully monitored clinical trial, 446 out of 450 skin tuberculosis patients treated with the Gerson diet recovered completely. He published articles in a dozen of the world's leading medical journals, establishing the Gerson treatment as the first cure for skin tuberculosis.

Dr. Gerson attracted the friendship of Nobel Prize winner Dr. Albert Schweitzer by curing Schweitzer's wife of lung tuberculosis after all conventional treatments had failed. Gerson and Schweitzer remained friends for life, and maintained regular correspondence. Dr. Schweitzer followed Gerson's progress as the dietary therapy was successfully applied to heart disease, kidney failure, and finally - cancer. Schweitzer's own Type II diabetes was cured by treatment with Gerson's therapy.

Today, Gerson Therapy is known as the most successful natural cancer treatment, and people from all over the world visit the Gerson Institute. The Therapy activates the body's extraordinary ability to heal itself through an organic, vegetarian diet, raw juices, coffee enemas and natural supplements. The Gerson Therapy treats the underlying causes of disease: toxicity and nutritional deficiency.

So, wait a minute. When was it discovered? In the 1920's? Oh. Soon, we are going to have the 100th Anniversary of the Gerson Therapy, and it's not on CNN?

It is probably not going to make it there, unless the Gerson Institute has a Coca-Cola budget to pay for a TV commercial. My experience of working in mainstream media, as a professional journalist and TV reporter, has been very eye-opening and disillusioning.

After my cancer disappeared from my four months of cleansing and fasting activities, I worked for several TV stations in Poland. I also wrote articles for magazines as a freelancer. I noticed that everything is sponsored. Even when it is not explicit, it is always somebody's PR campaign that stands to profit. There is no free media, just like there is no free lunch, and the mainstream media is definitely not going to bite the hand that's feeding it. Huge revenue from advertising and commercials come from pharmaceutical corporations who smear their brands and marketing tactics all over the screen and papers.

You need to learn to read between the lines. If information is presented to you, ask legitimate questions: Who paid for it? Who sponsored the research? Who is selling here? Who will profit from this news release? Space in magazines costs money. TV and radio time cost money. Internet ad campaigns cost money. Articles online cost money. Have no illusions. Read between the lines, just like you read labels on every single food product you put on your table. There is a multi-trillion dollar industry that profits on disinformation and disease.

A 22-year old Type II diabetic is worth three million dollars to the industry. He will be shooting insulin for life and his insurance will pay the bill. So, if you were selling insulin, why would you be interested in the curing and prevention of diabetes? That wouldn't compute in business. In fact, you would be invested in increasing your market share by lowering the age diabetes is being diagnosed. Is it surprising why so many kids nowadays are found obese and diabetic? Will they have to shoot insulin for the rest of their lives? How much are those children worth?

The same with cancer. The pharmaceutical cartels make more money on drugs addressing the side effects of chemotherapy than on chemotherapy itself. Perhaps, cancer is a brand? A brand of F.E.A.R. (False Evidence Appearing Real) Is this what we are being sold? Is this what we are buying?

A friend of mine, a very handsome man, was diagnosed with a throat cancer. He believes he got the HPV virus from giving oral pleasure to women. No one told him that if his blood were alkaline he wouldn't get any viruses in the first place, because viruses cannot live in an alkaline environment. No one told him that cancer thrives in an acidic environment and a shift in his blood pH could potentially cure him. He had surgery and 30 radiation procedures. His cancer was cured. He aged about 30 years and lost all his teeth. His case is considered a success. Today, a vaccine is administered to boys as a prevention against the virus. No change of diet recommended. Ever.

According to an article published in *JAMA (The Journal of American Medical Association)* by Dr. Barbara Starfield, the practice of medicine in hospitals is the third leading cause of death in America. The numbers she provided were based on conservative estimates.

In his article Death by Medicine, Gary Null, together with several other medical doctors, corrected her conservative estimates and made a complete listing of all the deaths that arise from medical treatment. He found that hospital medicine is the first leading cause of death, with over three-quarters of a million people dying every year:

"This fully referenced report shows the number of people having in-hospital, adverse reactions to prescribed drugs to be 2.2 million per year. The number of unnecessary antibiotics prescribed for viral infections is 20 million per year. The number of unnecessary medical and surgical procedures performed is 7.5 million per year. The number of people exposed to unnecessary hospitalization is 8.9 million per year.

The most stunning statistic, however, is that the total number of deaths caused by conventional medicine is an astounding 783,936 per year. It is now evident that the American medical system is the leading cause of death and injury in the US. (By contrast, the number of deaths attributable to heart disease in 2001 was 699,697, while the number of deaths attributable to cancer was 553,251)."

Imagine the number of people who died during the World Trade Center attack. That's the number of people dying in hospitals every week from *iatrogenesis* (death by doctor)!

Once, I wrote an article on the pharmaceutical industry. I interviewed Nobel Prize-winning doctors and researchers who are warning people about the dangers of the "business with disease". I also interviewed Wall Street brokers who explained to me the best pharmaceutical investments are drugs that "don't kill, don't cure and need to be taken chronically over a long period of time".

The corporations that own the patents on most of these products are economies the size of Switzerland. They sponsor charity concerts and cancer research foundations, and so on. Yet, given that they make trillions of dollars each year on the business of disease, you might ask if their incentives are lined up with our health.

One of the people I interviewed in my article was Dr. Matthias Rath, a medical doctor and researcher who worked with Nobel Prize winner Linus Pauling in his re-search on vitamin C. He calls this industry "the business with disease" and heads a huge media campaign for raising awareness about natural, holistic remedies that cause no harm to the body. Dr. Matthias Rath has the vision that the giant on clay legs will go bankrupt as we take back control over our health, instead of being medical victims.

Dr. Bruce Lipton, author of bestseller 'The Biology of Belief', points out that if Western medicine were based on scientific principles, it wouldn't be so lethal. He explains how medicine failed to catch up with cellular biology and is still stuck in the dogma of Genetic Determinism, and how it failed to apply the discoveries of quantum physics, and is still mis-grounded in the mechanistic world-view of Newtonian mechanics. Obviously, if the underlying premises of modern medicine are wrong, how could the scientific discoveries that stem from it be correct, and beneficial to the human body?

Bruce Lipton is one of the most inspiring scientists of our times. He dares to question the biases of contemporary science and observes how we bought into it:

"Science keeps trying to suggest that we are victims of everything, that cancer cells are victimizing us, or dis-eased cells are victimizing us, that bacteria can kill us; that we should be afraid of this and that, because we are these biochemical machines that are frail and Nature can override these machines.

"We feel victim to our genes and as a consequence we experience powerlessness, which is obviously very detrimental when trying to carry out our lives."

Above all, science has ignored the environment in which our body cells are swimming. Whether it is the emotional life of cancer patients, or their diet and lifestyle, or their relationships— at home and work.

When medical doctors today are speaking with a cancer patient, they're not putting into the equation that he or she is going through a divorce, or just lost a baby, or has lost trust in his partner, or is drowning in debt, or is living next to an electric power plant, etc. All these overwhelming situations don't matter a bit to Western medicine. Those are all factors drugs can't treat, so why bother?

You, however, can change them, if you only choose more for you, and acknowledge you create your life.

Medicine fails to ignore the blood pH of the patient, unless you find yourself in an emergency ambulance. Then they check your pH and they know if you are at 6, you are dead.

It amazes me how we can measure the pH of water in a fish tank and make sure it stays slightly alkaline so fungi won't overgrow and the fish won't get sick. It blows my mind how we keep our swimming pools in high pH while ignoring the pH of our bodies. The same standard of hygiene is not being applied to ourselves, leaving us susceptible to decay. On the contrary, we continue buying and drinking plastic bottled water, which is so acidic that you would do better not to drink it at all.

Doctors remain our magicians. Something magical happens when the doctor tells you that you are going to live. Something magical happens when the doctor tells you that you are going to die. The corporations are well aware of this magic and hire actors dressed as medical doctors to advertise drugs on tv. You can hire them too, for $5 on fiverr.com!

When a doctor tells you that you are going to die - if you buy into it - it can work like a death sentence that will kill your will - your life force. If your mind gives up, if your heart loses faith, so will your body, and it will slowly start shutting down.

I was very lucky to have been diagnosed first by a psychic, who told me I was going to live. I didn't believe a word she said. I thought she was crazy, and I wasn't going to do her fast, until a doctor confirmed I was ill. From then on, I never believed in a doctor. It was impossible to hypnotize me.

If that simple woman was able to see what was going on inside me with her intuition, then, Ladies and Gentlemen, What else is possible?

Many medical professionals, particularly nurses, are fully aware of the "business of disease", and they are eager to help people despite all the set up. After all, how can the patient get cured, when the health-care system is sick? Why would the doctor not send a patient for chemotherapy when he invested so many years in getting his degree, is still paying his medical school loans, has high liability insurance to pay each year, and may be profiting in yet other ways from following established systems?

I once met a Navy Medical Doctor. He was one of the most inspiring people I have ever met. He loves his job. Why? Because it's not a business for him. It's about helping the marines get their limbs back together. The creed at his Naval Hospital in Cherry Point, North Carolina, says: "Ensure Strength Through Caring." Too bad that motto is not universally upheld.

Another inspiring hero is Michael O'Doherty, who is a health pioneer and the founder of Plexus Bio-Energy. He is coming out with a family holistic health-care system.

His system represents the integration of a network of powerful and effective healing techniques that work by rebalancing the life energy within the body. The system has achieved exceptional results in the treatment of a wide range of conditions, often in cases that have proved difficult to treat by conventional means alone.

O'Doherty has had an enormous success in treating all sorts of incurable disorders. His touch-free energy healing modality has been featured on talk shows all over Ireland and in the USA. A number of celebrities attribute their recovery to his miraculous treatment, and people from all over the world come to learn his method. I have personally interviewed people who came out of wheelchairs and serious injuries, cured cancer, heart disease, asthma, Parkinson's, MS, and families whose children have been healed when doctors lost hope.

O'Doherty believes that your body is your business be-cause only you can control which thoughts, feelings and beliefs you allow into your brain, and those thoughts, beliefs, and feelings have been scientifically proven to significantly affect every cell in your body.

A former journalist, Michael O'Doherty is empowering people to take control over their health. He is all over the media saying:

"We cannot continue to treat disease in the same way we have been doing because it has failed; it's time for change."

According to Dr. Hulda Clark, a Canadian biologist and naturopath, author, and practitioner of alternative medicine, all human disease is related to parasitic infection. This makes total sense. The body fluids first become acidic in pH and then all sorts of fungi, microbes, and bacteria breed upon it. The problem starts when this entire parasitic zoo poops inside us. It is highly toxic to the human body and creates the environment that mutates cells. Interestingly enough, this process is reversible.

Dr. Robert O. Young, the author of the N.Y. Times bestseller, "The pH Miracle", has demonstrated on video a process called "pleomorphism" (many-formed) that occurs when a cell becomes cancerous and then becomes a healthy cell again, depending on its environment - the quality of fluids and energy that surround it. He measures the fluids with pH scale and the energy with MHz (megahertz: a unit of frequency, equal to one million cycles per second).

Young says our blood pH should be exactly 7.365, and demonstrates that a raw organic sprout is 250 MHz in foodfrequency, as opposed to a hamburger that barely scores 3 MHz.

It turns out that cancer begins when we have low pH levels in our blood and low MHz frequency in our food (less than 30 MHz). It is this low vibratory frequency of diet, emotions, and environment that breeds cancer.

Nature always claims her truth. Without mercy. No matter how many surgeries or chemotherapy treatments you may have, Nature always calls back. As Albert Einstein stated it - with no mercy: "The definition of insanity is to keep doing the same and expect a different result".

Of course, we are insane. We are constipated!!

The Bliss of Cancer

"No matter what you may be suffering from, regardless of how feverish, weak or desperately ill you may be, Nature wants to save you"

- Prof. Arnold Ehret

What if cancer is a wake up call to heal, awake, and choose a different lifestyle?

What if cancer is an invitation to step into leadership, inspiration and empowerment?

What if cancer is an opportunity for transformation?

My own self-healing journey has been led me to powerful discoveries in my life. I learned a lot about my body and got to know myself. I learned healing practices that have been available in different cultures for thousands of years, before Western medicine was invented. It led me to forgive my husband and develop a spiritual life of my own – a life of faith and trust that goes beyond the shackles of religion. It led me to enjoy my body, the gift of embodiment we all have as spiritual beings experiencing this physical reality. What an adventure that is! How could I be more grateful? How could I even possibly imagine cancer would lead me to travel all over the world, to touch the lives of so many people? And, surprisingly, I am not the only one who thinks cancer has led them to victory!

Every person I have interviewed who ever had cancer - whether cured naturally or treated with chemo - has told me: "It was the best thing that ever happened in my life. Paradoxically, it woke me up."

This awakening is a necessary part of healing. It is awakening to your dreams, to the biggest desires of your heart, to your greatness and to magic of the Universe. It is an awakening to life and you being unapologetically You.

Nothing does it so well as the realization you might die.

The possibility of death is actually thrilling. It's as close to life as it really gets. Of all the "deadlines" we have in our projects, death is the ultimate "deadline" on fulfilling life. Perhaps this is why in both Buddhist and Medieval civilizations monks had a creed of *memento mori*: "remember death". What if the awareness of death can actually make you fully alive?

People in the Western world avoid the notion of death, as a result hardly anyone is truly alive. They live in the denial as if nobody ever dies, everything is cool and we are all in the pursuit of eternal youth and happiness. Tralalala... Football, fast food, easy sex, and painkillers. Bigger car, bigger house. They are numbed not to notice how they age, get ill and dig themselves in debt. Men in particular like to create their wealth while destroying their health. Women trade their youth and beauty for security. In either case, cancer is a wake-up call.

My life has turned out to be blissful. The fat girl with an identity complex became an example of health, wellness and natural beauty. Ever since I cleansed and lost weight, I have received so much attention from men that at the beginning I had no idea how to handle it. I wasn't used to being considered attractive, for sure. I was shy, confused and almost scared. Before, I felt intimidated when I met a fit, healthy woman. I was afraid she would pass a judgement on me. Today, I am the one making conscious effort to reach out to women and help them. My body is fit, however I still look at the world through the eyes of the fat, sick and tired girl I once used to be. I remember how it feels.

My transformation came about so fast, I needed to actually hire a spiritual coach in order to sift out all the negative judgments I still kept having about myself - even though they were no longer relevant. My mind still continued to tell me lies: "I am fat. I am stupid. I am nothing." Something I kept saying daily during the crazy marriage that nearly killed me. The life coaching sessions opened my eyes to the world of energy and consciousness that has been truly healing me from inside out. I realized your body is only a 'hardware'. The software - your belief system is what runs it.

Your thoughts, feels and emotions are the operating system!

Today I know that the thoughts you are telling yourself can either kill you or heal you. It is the mind that creates the environment the body is bathing in. No matter what food you eat, if your mind is not set on joy, your body won't be fully alive.

Among all the research I came across, hardly anyone is studying the emotional life of cancer patients. What happened before they were found sick? What kind of events occurred, what kind of thoughts, feelings and emotions were going on inside them just before they were diagnosed?

I have interviewed a lot of people who had cancer. Most of them were female. I noticed women who had ovarian cancer were usually stuck in a marriage or a relationship where their man was not their partner but more like their child. They maintained this unauthentic relationship for many years sometimes and always reasoned their way back into it...

The body of the woman in those kinds of conditions develops tumors on the ovaries and makes her infertile. The body is consciously deciding: "We don't need a baby. We already have a baby!" (the partner). When staying in a co-dependent relationship, she keeps processing his moods and emotions, feels guilty for wanting to leave, she feels shame for having her own desires, and is often blamed for even attempting to take care of her own needs and foster her own dreams in life.

What if these emotions and judgments breed cancer? What if they somehow create an environment in the body that is toxic, and turns the body acidic and suicidal?

She doesn't know how to get out of this situation. She doesn't know how to leave. Divorce is despised in her religion, and Disney tales she was watching as a girl all ended with 'Happy

Ever After'. Music she hears on the radio keeps repeating the mantra: 'I love you. I can't live without you.' Insanity creeps in. The discrepancy between those tales and what she is actually experiencing in the relationship on daily basis is making her reality unbearable. She is haunted by his demons, and cancer is just a gateway - an suicidal escape route out of this madness.

A lot of women I interviewed who had breast cancer were suffering from chronic sadness. They were either considering themselves a victim of betrayal by their partner, family member, business associate, or they had lost a baby or a loved one. In every case there was some form of loss - loss of a person or loss of trust, and it perpetuated long-term sadness. Some of these women were sad for years.

I met some women with fibroids. Interestingly, all of them were breadwinners for their family. Their husbands were poets, artists, dreamers. Surprisingly, their relationships seemed to work. These women were making money, when the men were providing the inspiration. The only one that had to bend over to keep the balance of this equilibrium was the body. At moments, when the straw broke the camel's back, the entire uterus was removed, and the female would become even more masculine.

I am not a researcher, and definitely not a doctor. I am just a blonde asking questions: Why can't Western medicine seem to see the connection between lifestyle, emotions, and diet? Is it because it would require a serious interdisciplinary study? Would it not be worth it?

If cancer is a wake-up call, will you awaken now? If cancer is a gateway that can get you out of this world when you can no longer deal with it, ask the question: "What are you trying to get out of by creating cancer?"

Is it a unauthentic relationship or marriage, as it was in my case? Is it a humiliating job or overwhelming debts? Or maybe a family judgment passed onto you or by you? Maybe a family inheritance that was unfair and turned sour? Or a sense of boredom and lack of fulfillment in your life? A divorce that led to depression? Sexual abuse, years ago when you were little?

What are you trying to get out of by creating cancer?

We must have been insane to expect medical salvation from problems in our lives. Just as we are now insane in our lustful hopes that genetic engineering will save our planet and make us eternally healthy, young and sexy.

Instead of looking at the whole picture, instead of taking responsibility for the way we live our lives, we keep hoping scientists will discover a miracle cure, or quick-fix our DNA. The Human Genome Project demonstrated the human body cannot possibly be controlled by DNA, and even if it was, the question still would remain unanswered: If DNA controls life, what controls the DNA? If DNA is the software, who is the software Engineer?

Dr Bartlett, the author of "The Physics of Miracles" speculates on this subject:

"I think that perhaps our DNA is an antenna that picks up information from our environment, including our beliefs and our emotions. It then conveys that quantum potential to our bodies. When we unfold the imprinted information into our bioplasmic field, we then organize it into our bodies. We can literally manifest diseases in our bodies based or not based upon what we are congruent or not congruent with. To say this in another way, whatever we suppress will imprint into our morphic field, and be impressed onto our biology. That is why we really have to watch what we think."

In other words, we may think ourselves into a state of disease, or think ourselves into a state of wellness? Provided we do this thinking for long enough. This shifts our paradigm of health into the dimension of quantum physics and borderline miracles.

Is it possible that our medicine today is holding onto some outdated fairy-tales about Newtonian 'apples falling from the trees'? People used to believe the Earth was flat, and the man who said it wasn't, died at stake... Back then, the old world-view was upheld by the Vatican, today it is preached by Science and SienceFiction. Never the less, it is still outdated. And - it's dangerous to have wrong information.

If you met me before I healed, you would probably say: "She is just like her mom. She inherited the illness." As I am writing this book, my own mother is so sick. She has been dying for the past ten years or so. She is hospitalized every two weeks. She is not interested in getting healthy. Her husband (my father) for the first time is giving her all the attention she desires, and the whole family is giving her love. Finally. She is the center of attention she probably didn't get in her childhood, and definitely in her married life. There are absolutely no added benefits for my mother to getting well.

I have made different choices than my mom. I decided to do a lot of fresh juicing, take coffee enemas and leave toxic marriage. I decided not to settle for the kind of life she had endured. Best proof: life is not determined by DNA. Best proof: life is determined by your choice.

I noticed the craving for attention and the desire to be loved is one of the biggest things in the lives of people who have cancer. They crave love from people around them, and all of a sudden - if they have the diagnosis - they happen to get it. Finally. Instead of simply loving themselves, and caring for themselves, which would obviously reflect in choosing the healthiest lifestyle possible, they choose to get love in form of pity from others.

The biochemical rush sold to us as 'love' has nothing to do with love actually, and seems to be the hottest drug on the planet and definitely one of the most manipulative keywords. I see people stuck in hopeless relationships and marriages, even if it destroys their own mental and physical health, and financial wellbeing. My friend who is an ingenious psychologist in Los Angeles never accepts an invitation to attend a wedding or a funeral. He says: one leads to another.

The French say: *Je m'aime. J'adore moi-même. Je suis mon raison d' être.* I love me. I adore me. I am my own reason to be.

And, even though it sounds like a heresy, it is precisely the mantra that cured my Parisian friend of cancer after he was treated with chemotherapy twice. When he finally left his financially abusive relationship, and started to choose for himself, he healed, and cancer never came back.

Go ahead! You can create your own mantra! Imagine, what if there is no one else in the Universe but You? What if there is nothing else to crave? What if there is no energy to drain from anyone else? What if every person you meet is just another You? What if You are the love you desire?

Life is so beautiful, so real and so urgent. I would like to intoxicate you with aliveness. Instead of craving for love from this person or that person, what if you fall in choose to be authentic, present and fully alive? I guarantee you, life will claim you back immediately. Indeed. Go for a walk by yourself, and notice. Life is wooing you - with every leaf, every flower, every breeze, every ray of sunshine, every smile, every touch. You will feel life loving you back in every cell of your body, and you will be inspired to move, make love and dance.

Ever since I cured myself, I've been on the quest: What else is possible? What other limitations have I bought into? What other "walls" can I walk through? Ever since I healed and changed my life, I have fearlessly taken risks that are unheard of, and have been busy fulfilling my dreams.

As soon as I healed, I went for it. I applied for a job on tv. I got it the same day I had the interview: 'When do you want to start?' It came so easy and in my mind it was a very big deal all these years before I dared to show up. I interviewed leaders, politicians, celebrities, and I quickly noticed they have nothing new to say. I pulled out of mainstream media. Instead, I started to interview healers, shamans, psychics - people who had the gift just like Nadia. I spent years studying with them, attending workshops, healing sessions, and witnessing results that defy the limits of reason and appear to bend reality with the power of intention.

I know there are no victims in the world. There are only volunteers. We volunteer to forget who we are, to give up on life and surrender our power. We volunteer to buy into limiting points of view, limiting beliefs, and create our lives from limitation, trying to fit into a box. We volunteer to create disease and get out of this reality. Death or life are both choices.

How about you? Do you choose life? Do you love your life? The way it is. As it is.

Life is not a rehearsal. This is it. This is it.

The stage is ready. The Universe is watching. You are the great Artist, and the masterpiece you create is your Life. You are the Star. You write the script, you direct the show, you act in it, and you come to see it in the movie theatre. You even sell the tickets. It's always You.

How will you know you have fulfilled your life? What will convince you? What would you like to see in the world, when you take your flight? What if you own your life? And what if you give it away? How much are you going to gain? How much joy are you going to have?

MEET THE AUTHOR

Evita Ramparte is a Health Coach to Celebrities & CEOs, Business Mystic, and Force for Transformation. If you would like to join her community, get coaching or experience a retreat, visit her blog:

www.evitaramparte.com

www.ingramcontent.com/pod-product-compliance
Lightning Source LLC
Chambersburg PA
CBHW072147280526
45788CB00002B/791